W.B. SAUNDERS COMPANY
A Division of Elsevier Inc.

1600 John F. Kennedy Boulevard • Suite 1800 • Philadelphia, Pennsylvania 19103-2899

http://www.theclinics.com

ULTRASOUND CLINICS Volume 3, Number 4
October 2008 ISSN 1556-858X, ISBN-13: 978-1-4160-6364-3, ISBN-10: 1-4160-6364-1

Editor: Barton Dudlick
Developmental Editor: Theresa Collier

© **2008 Elsevier** ■ **All rights reserved.**

This journal and the individual contributions contained in it are protected under copyright by Elsevier, and the following terms and conditions apply to their use:

Photocopying
Single photocopies of single articles may be made for personal use as allowed by national copyright laws. Permission of the Publisher and payment of a fee is required for all other photocopying, including multiple or systematic copying, copying for advertising or promotional purposes, resale, and all forms of document delivery. Special rates are available for educational institutions that wish to make photocopies for non-profit educational classroom use. For information on how to seek permission visit www.elsevier.com/permissions or call: (+44) 1865 843830 (UK)/ (+1) 215 239 3804 (USA).

Derivative Works
Subscribers may reproduce tables of contents or prepare lists of articles including abstracts for internal circulation within their institutions. Permission of the Publisher is required for resale or distribution outside the institution. Permission of the Publisher is required for all other derivative works, including compilations and translations (please consult www.elsevier.com/permissions).

Electronic Storage or Usage
Permission of the Publisher is required to store or use electronically any material contained in this journal, including any article or part of an article (please consult www.elsevier.com/permissions). Except as outlined above, no part of this publication may be reproduced, stored in a retrieval system or transmitted in any form or by any means, electronic, mechanical, photocopying, recording or otherwise, without prior written permission of the Publisher.

Notice
No responsibility is assumed by the Publisher for any injury and/or damage to persons or property as a matter of products liability, negligence or otherwise, or from any use or operation of any methods, products, instructions or ideas contained in the material herein. Because of rapid advances in the medical sciences, in particular, independent verification of diagnoses and drug dosages should be made.

Although all advertising material is expected to conform to ethical (medical) standards, inclusion in this publication does not constitute a guarantee or endorsement of the quality or value of such product or of the claims made of it by its manufacturer.

Ultrasound Clinics (ISSN 1556-858X) is published quarterly by W.B. Saunders, 360 Park Avenue South, New York, NY 10010-1710. Months of publication are January, April, July, and October. Business and editorial offices: 1600 John F. Kennedy Boulevard, Suite 1800, Philadelphia, Pennsylvania 19103-2899. Accounting and circulation offices: 6277 Sea Harbor Drive, Orlando, FL 32887-4800. Periodicals postage paid at New York NY, and additional mailing offices. Subscription prices are $189 per year for (US individuals), $274 per year for (US institutions), $94 per year for (US students and residents), $215 per year for (Canadian individuals), $306 per year for (Canadian institutions), $229 per year for (international individuals), $306 per year for (international institutions), and $114 per year for (Canadian and foreign students/residents). To receive student/resident rate, orders must be accompanied by name of affiliated institution, date of term, and the signature of program/residency coordinator on institution letterhead. Orders will be billed at individual rate until proof of status is received. Foreign air speed delivery is included in all Clinics subscription prices. All prices are subject to change without notice. **POSTMASTER:** Send address changes to *Ultrasound Clinics*, Elsevier Periodicals Customer Service, 11830 Westline Industrial Drive, St. Louis, MO 63146. **Customer Service: 1-800-654-2452 (US). From outside the United States, call 1-314-453-7041. Fax: 1-314-453-5170.** E-mail: JournalsCustomerService-usa@elsevier.com (for print support) or JournalsOnlineSupport-usa@elsevier.com (for online support).

Reprints: For copies of 100 or more, of articles in this publication, please contact the Commercial Reprints Department, Elsevier Inc., 360 Park Avenue South, New York, NY 10010-1710. Tel.: (+1) 212-633-3812; Fax: (+1) 212-462-1935; E-mail: reprints@elsevier.com.

Printed in the United States of America.

SCANNED
JAN 0 5 2009

Advanced Obstetrical Ultrasound: Fetal Brain, Spine, and Limb Abnormalities

Guest Editors

NOAM LAZEBNIK, MD
ROEE S. LAZEBNIK, MD, PhD

ULTRASOUND CLINICS

www.ultrasound.theclinics.com

SAUNDERS an imprint of ELSEVIER, Inc.

W.B. SAUNDERS COMPANY
A Division of Elsevier Inc.

1600 John F. Kennedy Boulevard • Suite 1800 • Philadelphia, Pennsylvania 19103-2899

http://www.theclinics.com

ULTRASOUND CLINICS Volume 3, Number 4
October 2008 ISSN 1556-858X, ISBN-13: 978-1-4160-6364-3, ISBN-10: 1-4160-6364-1

Editor: Barton Dudlick
Developmental Editor: Theresa Collier

© **2008 Elsevier** ■ **All rights reserved.**

This journal and the individual contributions contained in it are protected under copyright by Elsevier, and the following terms and conditions apply to their use:

Photocopying
Single photocopies of single articles may be made for personal use as allowed by national copyright laws. Permission of the Publisher and payment of a fee is required for all other photocopying, including multiple or systematic copying, copying for advertising or promotional purposes, resale, and all forms of document delivery. Special rates are available for educational institutions that wish to make photocopies for non-profit educational classroom use. For information on how to seek permission visit www.elsevier.com/permissions or call: (+44) 1865 843830 (UK)/ (+1) 215 239 3804 (USA).

Derivative Works
Subscribers may reproduce tables of contents or prepare lists of articles including abstracts for internal circulation within their institutions. Permission of the Publisher is required for resale or distribution outside the institution. Permission of the Publisher is required for all other derivative works, including compilations and translations (please consult www.elsevier.com/permissions).

Electronic Storage or Usage
Permission of the Publisher is required to store or use electronically any material contained in this journal, including any article or part of an article (please consult www.elsevier.com/permissions). Except as outlined above, no part of this publication may be reproduced, stored in a retrieval system or transmitted in any form or by any means, electronic, mechanical, photocopying, recording or otherwise, without prior written permission of the Publisher.

Notice
No responsibility is assumed by the Publisher for any injury and/or damage to persons or property as a matter of products liability, negligence or otherwise, or from any use or operation of any methods, products, instructions or ideas contained in the material herein. Because of rapid advances in the medical sciences, in particular, independent verification of diagnoses and drug dosages should be made.

Although all advertising material is expected to conform to ethical (medical) standards, inclusion in this publication does not constitute a guarantee or endorsement of the quality or value of such product or of the claims made of it by its manufacturer.

Ultrasound Clinics (ISSN 1556-858X) is published quarterly by W.B. Saunders, 360 Park Avenue South, New York, NY 10010-1710. Months of publication are January, April, July, and October. Business and editorial offices: 1600 John F. Kennedy Boulevard, Suite 1800, Philadelphia, Pennsylvania 19103-2899. Accounting and circulation offices: 6277 Sea Harbor Drive, Orlando, FL 32887-4800. Periodicals postage paid at New York NY, and additional mailing offices. Subscription prices are $189 per year for (US individuals), $274 per year for (US institutions), $94 per year for (US students and residents), $215 per year for (Canadian individuals), $306 per year for (Canadian institutions), $229 per year for (international individuals), $306 per year for (international institutions), and $114 per year for (Canadian and foreign students/residents). To receive student/resident rate, orders must be accompanied by name of affiliated institution, date of term, and the signature of program/residency coordinator on institution letterhead. Orders will be billed at individual rate until proof of status is received. Foreign air speed delivery is included in all Clinics subscription prices. All prices are subject to change without notice. **POSTMASTER:** Send address changes to *Ultrasound Clinics*, Elsevier Periodicals Customer Service, 11830 Westline Industrial Drive, St. Louis, MO 63146. **Customer Service: 1-800-654-2452 (US). From outside the United States, call 1-314-453-7041. Fax: 1-314-453-5170. E-mail: JournalsCustomerService-usa@elsevier.com (for print support) or JournalsOnlineSupport-usa@elsevier.com (for online support).**

Reprints: For copies of 100 or more, of articles in this publication, please contact the Commercial Reprints Department, Elsevier Inc., 360 Park Avenue South, New York, NY 10010-1710. Tel.: (+1) 212-633-3812; Fax: (+1) 212-462-1935; E-mail: reprints@elsevier.com.

Printed in the United States of America.

Contributors

GUEST EDITORS

NOAM LAZEBNIK, MD
Associate Professor of OBGYN, Medical Genetics, and Radiology Department of Obstetrics and Gynecology, Case Western Reserve University, University Hospitals of Cleveland, Cleveland, Ohio

ROEE S. LAZEBNIK, MD, PhD
Siemens Healthcare Ultrasound Business Unit, Mountain View, California

AUTHORS

JACQUES S. ABRAMOWICZ, MD
Francis T. & Lester B. Knight Professor of Obstetrics & Gynecology; Director, Ob/Gyn Ultrasound, Department of Obstetrics and Gynecology; and Co-director, Rush Fetal and Neonatal Medicine Program, Rush University Medical Center, Chicago, Illinois

ERAN BORNSTEIN, MD
Division of Maternal Fetal Medicine, Department of Obstetrics & Gynecology, NYU School of Medicine, New York, New York

DAVID CHITAYAT, MD
Head, The Prenatal Diagnosis and Medical Genetics Program, Mount Sinai Hospital; Department of Obstetrics and Gynecology, Mount Sinai Hospital; and The Hospital for Sick Children, Division of Clinical and Metabolic Genetics, University of Toronto, Toronto, Ontario, Canada

ORIT A. GLENN, MD
Associate Professor of Clinical Radiology and Neurosurgery, Department of Radiology, Diagnostic Neuroradiology, University of California, San Francisco, California

ARIE KOIFMAN
The Prenatal Diagnosis and Medical Genetics Program, Mount Sinai Hospital; Department of Obstetrics and Gynecology, Mount Sinai Hospital; and The Hospital for Sick Children, Division of Clinical and Metabolic Genetics, University of Toronto, Toronto, Ontario, Canada

NOAM LAZEBNIK, MD
Associate Professor of OBGYN, Medical Genetics, and Radiology Department of Obstetrics and Gynecology, Case Western Reserve University, University Hospitals of Cleveland, Cleveland, Ohio

TALLY LERMAN-SAGIE, MD
Director, Pediatric Neurology Unit, Edith Wolfson Medical Center, Holon; Associated Professor, Sackler School of Medicine, Tel-Aviv University, Tel-Aviv, Israel

GUSTAVO MALINGER, MD
Director, Prenatal Diagnosis Unit, Department of Obstetrics and Gynecology, Edith Wolfson Medical Center, Holon, Israel; Senior Lecturer, Sackler School of Medicine, Tel-Aviv University, Tel-Aviv, Israel

ANA MONTEAGUDO, MD, RDMS
Professor of Obstetrics & Gynecology, Division of Maternal Fetal Medicine, Department of Obstetrics & Gynecology, NYU School of Medicine, New York, New York

ORI NEVO, MD
Department of Obstetrics and Gynecology, Sunnybrook Health Sciences Centre, University of Toronto, Toronto, Ontario, Canada

RITSUKO K. POOH, MD, PhD
(CRIFM) Clinical Research Institute of Fetal Medicine PMC, Uehommachi, Tennoji, Osaka, Japan

Contributors

EDGARDO CORRAL SEREÑO, MD
Director, Unidad de Ultrasonografia y Medicina Fetal, Servicio de Obsteticia y Ginecologia, Hospital Regional, Rancagua, Chile

EYAL SHEINER, MD, PhD
Senior Lecturer, Department of Obstetrics & Gynecology, Soroka University Medical Center, Ben Gurion University of the Negev, Beer Sheva, Israel

ALICE B. SMITH, LT. COL, USAF, MC
Chief, Neuroradiology, Department of Radiologic Pathology, Armed Forces Institute of Pathology, Washington; and Assistant Professor, Department of Radiology and Radiological Sciences, Uniformed Services University of the Health Sciences, Bethesda, Maryland

ILAN E. TIMOR-TRITSCH, MD, RDMS
Professor of Obstetrics & Gynecology, Division of Ultrasound in Obstetrics & Gynecology, Department of Obstetrics & Gynecology, NYU School of Medicine, New York, New York

ANTS TOI
Department of Diagnostic Imaging, Mount Sinai Hospital, University of Toronto, Toronto, Ontario, Canada

Contents

Preface ix

Noam Lazebnik and Roee S. Lazebnik

The Utilization of Three and Four Dimensional Technology in Fetal Neurosonology 489

Eran Bornstein, Ana Monteagudo, and Ilan E. Timor-Tritsch

> This article discusses the clinical use of three-dimensional technology while performing a fetal neuroscan. This technique allows us to better define the spatial relationship of brain structures and possible malformations. The varieties of display modes and the infinite number of different planes that can be generated facilitate the diagnostic process. Additional values of this technology include an off-line analysis of the volume by the sonographer or sonologist to obtain the necessary planes, as well as an electronic transmittal for an off-site expert to provide a second opinion consultation. This modality requires a short acquisition time, allowing high patient through-put and increased patient satisfaction. In addition, it is an excellent teaching tool and provides valuable information to consulting such experts as pediatric surgeons, plastic surgeons, neonatologists, neurologists and neurosurgeons.

3-D and 4-D Fetal Neuroscan: Sharing the Know-how and Tricks of the Trade 517

Eran Bornstein, Ana Monteagudo, and Ilan E. Timor-Tritsch

> Visual information from 2-D images may be limited in reflecting a 3-D structural reality. 3-D techniques have emerged enabling acquisition of an entire volume of spatial ultrasound information that can be analyzed and displayed in multiple planes and display modes that exceed the capacities of 2-D US and better reflect the 3-D nature of a structure or anomaly. In the future 3-D evaluation of the fetal body will be an inherent part of fetal study in cases of congenital anomaly, specifically fetal brain abnormality. This article focuses on the technique for obtaining and analyzing acquired volumes and displaying them.

The Utility of Volume Sonography for the Detection of Fetal Spine Abnormalities 529

Noam Lazebnik, Eran Bornstein, and Ilan E. Timor-Tritsch

> Sonographic evaluation of the fetal vertebral column is essential for fetal central nervous system evaluation and valuable for ruling out genetic conditions. This article provides an overview for obtaining and manipulating fetal vertebrae three-dimensional data as to obtain the necessary diagnostic views. Additional technical information is provided elsewhere in this issue. This discussion is limited to include only the most common fetal vertebral abnormalities. The same technical principals, however, enable detection of many additional abnormalities.

Fetal Neuroimaging of Neural Migration Disorder 541

Ritsuko K. Pooh

> Prenatal diagnosis of migration disorder is among the most difficult challenges of an antenatal sonographic examination. Anterior coronal demonstration of the sylvian fissures

is recommended as the screening of cortical development and maldevelopment. Once suspicion of a migration disorder develops, MR imaging is the preferred modality for demonstration of cortical development. Considering that migration disorders occur before fetal viability but detection of brain lesions is most commonly performed in the third trimester, this presents a diagnostic dilemma. Early detection of migration disorder with severe prognosis is among the central missions of fetal neuroimaging.

The Differential Diagnosis of Fetal Intracranial Cystic Lesions 553
Gustavo Malinger, Edgardo Corral Sereño, and Tally Lerman-Sagie

Fetal Intracranial cysts can be diagnosed during pregnancy by the use of ultrasound scan. The cysts can be found in different brain compartments and may be of diverse origins. Choroid plexus and arachnoid cysts are the most commonly diagnosed lesions and when isolated carry a good prognosis. Intraparenchymal cysts may have different etiologies, and the prognosis depends largely on the location and the extent of the lesion.

Magnetic Resonance Imaging Following Suspicion for Fetal Brain Anomalies 559
Alice B. Smith and Orit A. Glenn

Fetal MR imaging provides a useful adjunct in the evaluation of anomalies of the fetal brain noted on ultrasound. The higher resolution of fetal MR imaging allows for improved assessment of cortical malformations and other anomalies. The use of fetal MR imaging is relatively new, however, and understanding of the imaging findings continues to evolve. In addition, the improvement of newer techniques, such as diffusion weighted MR imaging, should lead to improved understanding of the developing fetal brain and the impact of ischemic, infectious, and developmental insults.

Ultrasound of the Fetal Cranium: Review of Current Literature 583
Eyal Sheiner and Jacques S. Abramowicz

Fetal cranial defects and abnormal skull shape are amenable to ultrasound study diagnosis. Correct identification of the nature of the abnormality is extremely important and helpful in establishing diagnosis and longterm prognosis. In addition it might direct the care provider to apply the correct genetic study, chromosome or DNA related, for final diagnosis confirmation. This article discusses normal and abnormal fetal skull anatomy as observed using ultrasound technology.

Diagnostic Approach to Prenatally Diagnosed Limb Abnormalities 595
Arie Koifman, Ori Nevo, Ants Toi, and David Chitayat

Limb formation occurs at 4–12 weeks gestation and involves many genes and gene families. The prevalence of limb abnormalities is approximately 6/10,000 live births, with higher incidence in the upper limbs compared to the lower limbs (3.4/10,000 and 1.1/10,000 respectively). Limb abnormalities are morphologically and etiologically heterogenous group of abnormalities and most are amenable for prenatal diagnosis. The investigation and counselling of woman/couple with prenatally diagnosed fetal limb abnormality requires a multidisciplinary team including obstetrician, radiologist, clinical geneticist, neonatologist/pediatrician and a pediatric orthopedic surgeon. Other specialties may be needed if other abnormalities are detected.

Index 609

Ultrasound Clinics

FORTHCOMING ISSUES

January 2009

US-Guided Interventions
Hishan Tchelepi, MD, *Guest Editor*

April 2009

Advanced in Ultrasound
Vikram S. Dogra, MD, *Guest Editor*

RECENT ISSUES

July 2008

Women's Imaging
Vikram S. Dogra, MD, and Deniz Akata, MD, *Guest Editors*

April 2008

Ophthalmologic Ultrasound
Arun D. Singh, MD, Brandy C. Hayden, BS, and Charles J. Pavlin, MD, *Guest Editors*

RELATED INTEREST

January 2008
Radiologic Clinics of North America
Genitourinary Tract Imaging
Michael A. Blake, MRCPI, and Mannudeep K. Kalra, MD, *Guest Editors*

May 2007
Radiologic Clinics of North America
Emergency Cross-Sectional Imaging
Vikram S. Dogra, MD, and Shweta Bhatt, MD, *Guest Editors*

THE CLINICS ARE NOW AVAILABLE ONLINE!

Access your subscription at:
www.theclinics.com

GOAL STATEMENT

The goal of the *Ultrasound Clinics* is to keep practicing radiologists and radiology residents up to date with current clinical practice in ultrasound by providing timely articles reviewing the state of the art in patient care.

ACCREDITATION

The *Ultrasound Clinics* is planned and implemented in accordance with the Essential Areas and Policies of the Accreditation Council for Continuing Medical Education (ACCME) through the joint sponsorship of the University of Virginia School of Medicine and Elsevier. The University of Virginia School of Medicine is accredited by the ACCME to provide continuing medical education for physicians.

The University of Virginia School of Medicine designates this educational activity for a maximum of 15 *AMA PRA Category 1 Credits*™. Physicians should only claim credit commensurate with the extent of their participation in the activity.

The American Medical Association has determined that physicians not licensed in the US who participate in this CME activity are eligible for 15 *AMA PRA Category 1 Credits*™.

Credit can be earned by reading the text material, taking the CME examination online at http://www.theclinics.com/home/cme, and completing the evaluation. After taking the test, you will be required to review any and all incorrect answers. Following completion of the test and evaluation, your credit will be awarded and you may print your certificate.

FACULTY DISCLOSURE/CONFLICT OF INTEREST

The University of Virginia School of Medicine, as an ACCME accredited provider, endorses and strives to comply with the Accreditation Council for Continuing Medical Education (ACCME) Standards of Commercial Support, Commonwealth of Virginia statutes, University of Virginia policies and procedures, and associated federal and private regulations and guidelines on the need for disclosure and monitoring of proprietary and financial interests that may affect the scientific integrity and balance of content delivered in continuing medical education activities under our auspices.

The University of Virginia School of Medicine requires that all CME activities accredited through this institution be developed independently and be scientifically rigorous, balanced and objective in the presentation/discussion of its content, theories and practices.

All authors/editors participating in an accredited CME activity are expected to disclose to the readers relevant financial relationships with commercial entities occurring within the past 12 months (such as grants or research support, employee, consultant, stock holder, member of speakers bureau, etc.). The University of Virginia School of Medicine will employ appropriate mechanisms to resolve potential conflicts of interest to maintain the standards of fair and balanced education to the reader. Questions about specific strategies can be directed to the Office of Continuing Medical Education, University of Virginia School of Medicine, Charlottesville, Virginia.

The faculty and staff of the University of Virginia Office of Continuing Medical Education have no financial affiliations to disclose.

The authors/editors listed below have identified no professional or financial affiliations for themselves or their spouse/partner:

Matthew J. Bassignani, MD (Test Author); Eran Bornstein, MD; David Chitayat, MD; Barton Dudlick (Acquisitions Editor); Orit A. Glenn, MD; Arie Koifman, MD; Noem Lazebnik, MD (Guest Editor); Tally Lerman-Sagie, MD; Gustavo Malinger, MD; Ana Monteagudo, MD, RDMS; Ori Nevo, MD; Ritsuko K. Pooh, MD, PhD; Edguardo Corral Sereño, MD; Eyal Sheiner, MD, PhD; Alice Boyd Smith, MD, Lt. Col, USAF, MC; and Ilan E. Timor-Tritsch, MD, RDMS.

The authors/editors listed below have identified the following professional or financial affiliations for themselves or their spouse/partner:

Jacques S. Abramowicz, MD is a consultant for Philips Medical and conducts research for Zonare.
Roee S. Lazebik, MD, PhD (Guest Editor) is employed by Siemens Healthcare Ultrasound Business Unit.

Disclosure of Discussion of Non-FDA Approved Uses for Pharmaceutical Products and/or Medical Devices.
The University of Virginia School of Medicine, as an ACCME provider, requires that all faculty presenters identify and disclose any off-label uses for pharmaceutical and medical device products. The University of Virginia School of Medicine recommends that each physician fully review all the available data on new products or procedures prior to clinical use.

TO ENROLL

To enroll in the Ultrasound Clinics Continuing Medical Education program, call customer service at 1-800-654-2452 or visit us online at www.theclinics.com/home/cme. The CME program is available to subscribers for an additional fee of $205.00.

Preface

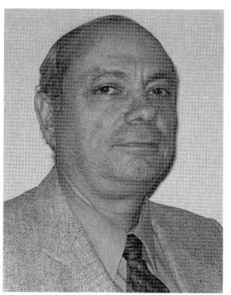
Noam Lazebnik, MD

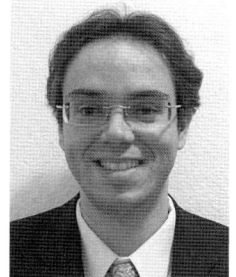
Roee S. Lazebnik, MD, PhD

Guest Editors

Ultrasound imaging is relatively inexpensive, safe, real-time, and readily available in hospitals and clinics throughout the world. For almost forty years, sonography progressed steadily with advances in both clinical application and equipment performance. It is truly an indispensable tool in obstetrics for the diagnosis and management of many diseases, encompassing three generations of women and millions of studies.

At a given time, many new areas of ultrasound imaging are under development and investigation. Of these, volumetric ultrasound (three-dimensional [3D]/four-dimensional [4D] US) generated particularly great interest by the clinical community. Yet, despite decades of exploration, only during the past five years has volume sonography advanced to a practical state for routine diagnostic and interventional applications. Recent advances in computer technology and visualization techniques allow real-time reconstruction, visualization, and manipulation of volume data using inexpensive desktop computers. These continue to enable many physicians to explore the full potential of this modality for a variety of diagnostic and therapeutic applications.

The most clinically mature applications for volume ultrasound technology are within the realm of obstetrics. Often, a volume approach provides information that is not readily available using conventional two-dimensional (2D) imaging. Volume or surface rendering, coupled with multiplanner reformatted displays, allow a comprehensive review of fetal organs and skeleton. The ability to rapidly reorient the active view for optimal visualization of the target anatomy permits rapid identification of normal and abnormal structures. Numerous studies demonstrate the utility of volume ultrasound in obstetrics, often citing advantages compared with conventional 2D ultrasound. These include improved comprehension of fetal anatomy by the parents, allowing more informed decisions for management of the pregnancy; improved maternal/fetal bonding due to intuitive visualization of fetal features; improved identification of fetal anomalies; and greater accuracy in volume measurements to determine the size and extent of anomalies.

In this issue of *Ultrasound Clinics*, Bornstein and colleagues extensively review the technical and clinical aspects of performing a fetal neuroscan. The interested reader is referred to practical advice on imaging-based techniques and investigations, a comprehensive review by Pilu and colleagues, for additional information.[1] In another article, Lazebnik and coauthors discuss the utilization and advantages of 3D ultrasound technology in the evaluation of normal and common congenital spine and vertebral anomalies.

Proper diagnosis of congenital brain anomalies is challenging, even with the use of modern sonographic equipment. A high level of skill and expertise, as well as an understanding of the nature of the abnormality, are of utmost importance. Imaging-based information may drive the choice of prenatal testing (chromosome, DNA, culture). Prenatal diagnosis of neuronal migration disorders, while difficult, is possible using antenatal diagnostic sonography. Dr. Ritsuko Pooh, a leading researcher of sonographic fetal brain imaging, discusses neuronal migration disorders caused by the abnormal migration of neurons in the developing brain and nervous system. These include focal cerebrocortical dysgenesis, heterotopia, polymicrogyria, lissencephaly or pachygyria, and schizencephaly.

Intracranial cystic lesions are frequently diagnosed using fetal ultrasound. Although the most prevalent cysts are benign (choroid plexus and arachnoid cysts), the mere suspicion of a brain lesion during fetal life raises serious concerns for the prospective parents regarding the neurodevelopmental outcome of their child. Malinger and colleagues review the diagnostic approach and particularly the differential diagnosis and prognosis of intracranial cystic lesions identified in utero in the context of prenatal counseling.

Although fetal ultrasound is considered the standard of care in the evaluation of fetal anomalies, an understanding of the technology's limitations is important. These limitations include decreased visibility of fetal structures due to maternal body habitus, position of the fetal head, ossification of the fetal skull, and, in some cases, oligohydramnios. Fetal MR imaging is applied by many medical centers in addition to ultrasound in an attempt to further enhance the antenatal diagnostic process. The utilization of fetal brain MR imaging is discussed by Smith and Glenn, and is particularly helpful in the diagnosis of anomalies of sulcation, periventricular nodular heterotopia, callosal agenesis, periventricular white matter injury, cerebellar dysplasia, germinal matrix, and intraventricular hemorrhage during the second and third trimesters. This approach provides additional information for prenatal counseling and delivery planning.

Anomalies of the fetal brain are relatively common and have the potential to result in severe morbidity or mortality. Though much has been published regarding the fetal brain, less has been discussed about the fetal skull. Images of the fetal skull are routinely obtained during ultrasound examination. The frontal, parietal, thin squama of the temporal bones and occipital bones, which together form the calvaria, are visualized. The cartilaginous zones of articulation of these bones—the coronal, sagittal, and lamboid sutures—are visible, as well as the fontanelles (mainly the anterior and the posterior). By combining 2D multiplanner display and 3D-rendered images in the maximum mode, the various bones and sutures of the skull are clearly defined. The article by Sheiner and Abramowicz discusses the sonographic features of the normal and abnormal fetal skull utilizing 2D and 3D ultrasound technologies.

Fetal limb abnormalities are of utmost importance for prenatal diagnosis of fetal disorders and appropriate genetic counseling. Limb abnormalities may be isolated or found in association with other abnormalities. These may result from malformations, deformations, or disruptions, as well as a part of a dysplasia such as skeletal dysplasia. Sonographic image quality depends on many factors, including the patient's body habitus, quality of the ultrasound equipment, and operator skill. The article by Koifman and coworkers reviews a methodical approach to imaging the fetus with prenatally diagnosed limb abnormalities. This process enables the medical team to provide the mother and the family with information regarding the nature of the abnormality, differential diagnosis, prognosis, and management options.

Overall, ultrasound is an established and continually evolving modality for the evaluation of the fetus across many organ systems. As ultrasound technology evolves, so does our understanding of the diagnostic information it provides. We also continue to discover new techniques for image acquisition and methods for data manipulation. Ultimately, these developments lead to increased diagnostic confidence and thus benefit both patients and clinicians.

Noam Lazebnik, MD
Department of Obstetrics and Gynecology
University Hospitals of Cleveland
11100 Euclid Avenue
Cleveland, OH 44060, USA

Roee S. Lazebnik, MD, PhD
Siemens Healthcare
Ultrasound Business Unit
1230 Shore Bird Way
Mountain View, CA 94043, USA

E-mail addresses:
noam.lazebnik@uhhospitals.org (N. Lazebnik)
roee.lazebnik@siemens.com (R.S. Lazebnik)

REFERENCE

1. Pilu G, Ghi T, Carletti A, et al. Three-dimensional ultrasound examination of the fetal central nervous system. Ultrasound in Obstetrics and Gynecology 2007;30(2):233–45.

The Utilization of 3D and 4D Technology in Fetal Neurosonology

Eran Bornstein, MD*, Ana Monteagudo, MD, RDMS, Ilan E. Timor-Tritsch, MD, RDMS

KEYWORDS

- 3D ultrasound • Brain anomaly
- Fetal brain • Neuroscan • Volume manipulation

This article discusses the clinical use of three-dimensional (3D) technology while performing a fetal neuroscan. Before reading this article, one should first be familiar with the technical aspects of performing this type of fetal study. For complete details and comprehensive discussion of the advantages of 3D technique as well as technical aspects of obtaining quality volume data and subsequently displaying quality images, the reader is referred to "3D and 4D Fetal Neuroscan: Sharing the Know-how and Tricks of the Trade" by Bornstein and colleagues in this issue of the Clinics.

HOW TO PERFORM THE 3D FETAL NEUROSCAN
Volume Acquisition

To perform fetal neuroscan, either the transabdominal or the transvaginal approach should be instituted.[1–4] The authors' preference, if fetal position permits, is the transvaginal approach, using a high-frequency probe aligned with the fontanelle when possible or the sagittal or coronal sutures. **Fig. 1** displays a surface rendering of the fetal scull demonstrating the acoustic window, which is consistent with the anterior fontanelle and the sutures. After identification of the anterior fontanelle or the superior sagittal sinus, an adequate 2D-transvaginal picture of the fetal brain is obtained (**Fig. 2**). The fetal head may be gently manipulated and controlled by the examiner's free hand to perfectly align the footprint of the probe with a fontanelle or a suture. Once the ultrasound beam has been aligned with the longitudinal axis of the fetal brain through the anterior fontanelle or the sagittal suture, and a clear and diagnostically good 2D image of the fetal brain is seen, the brain volume can be acquired in the sagittal plane. A second volume should be obtained in the coronal plane by rotating the probe 90° from the median section of the fetal brain. These two volumes should be acquired using a 60° to 80° angle width to include the whole fetal brain in the volume. The quality of the image depends on the acquisition speed. The authors' usually prefer slow acquisition speed, yielding a more detailed volume for imaging the fetal brain. Fast acquisition using the low or medium resolution is more adequate for acquiring volumes from a moving fetus. When the transvaginal approach is not possible, the transabdominal approach is used to obtain two acquisitions in two perpendicular planes. As the sagittal plane is usually hard to obtain transabdominally, the volume should be acquired in both the axial and the coronal planes. The authors usually acquire the volume with a mechanical sweep of a 45° angle width during the second trimester scan. With advanced gestational age during the third trimester, the angle width should be increased to about 60° to include the entire brain in the acquired volume.[5]

Orientation within the Volume

Now that the volume has been acquired, the authors' protocol is to first manipulate the volume to

---

Division of Maternal Fetal Medicine, Department of Obstetrics & Gynecology, New York University School of Medicine, 550 First Avenue, Room 9N26, New York, NY 10016, USA
* Corresponding author.
E-mail address: eranbor@yahoo.com (E. Bornstein).

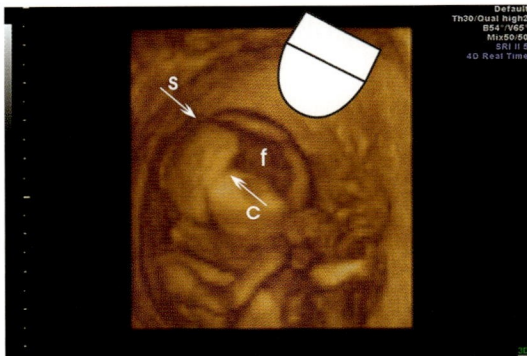

Fig. 1. The cranial bone is seen in this 3D surface rendering of the fetal scalp demonstrating the coronal (c) and sagittal (s) sutures, as well as the anterior fontanelle (f), which serves as a large acoustic window in this 15-postmenstrual week's fetus. The vaginal probe should be directed toward the fontanelle to enable a high-resolution fetal neuroscan. The sagittal and coronal suture may also be used if fetal position does not facilitate the transfontanelle approach.

a "starting position" so it is always displayed in the same orientation in the multiplanar display boxes:

The authors' protocol consists of manipulating the volume so that the coronal plane is displayed in Box "A," the sagittal plane in Box "B" and the axial plane in Box "C." Box B should display the fetal head in the sagittal plane when the fetus "looks" to the left of the screen. This way, in the coronal image in Box A, the right and left sides will be displayed as in traditional imaging. In Box C, the forehead will be on the bottom. **Fig. 3** demonstrates a multiplanar display of the fetal after the initial acquisition (before manipulation). The arrows mark the manipulations, which were required and the order in which they were performed to position the volume in the correct orientation in the three orthogonal planes, as is shown

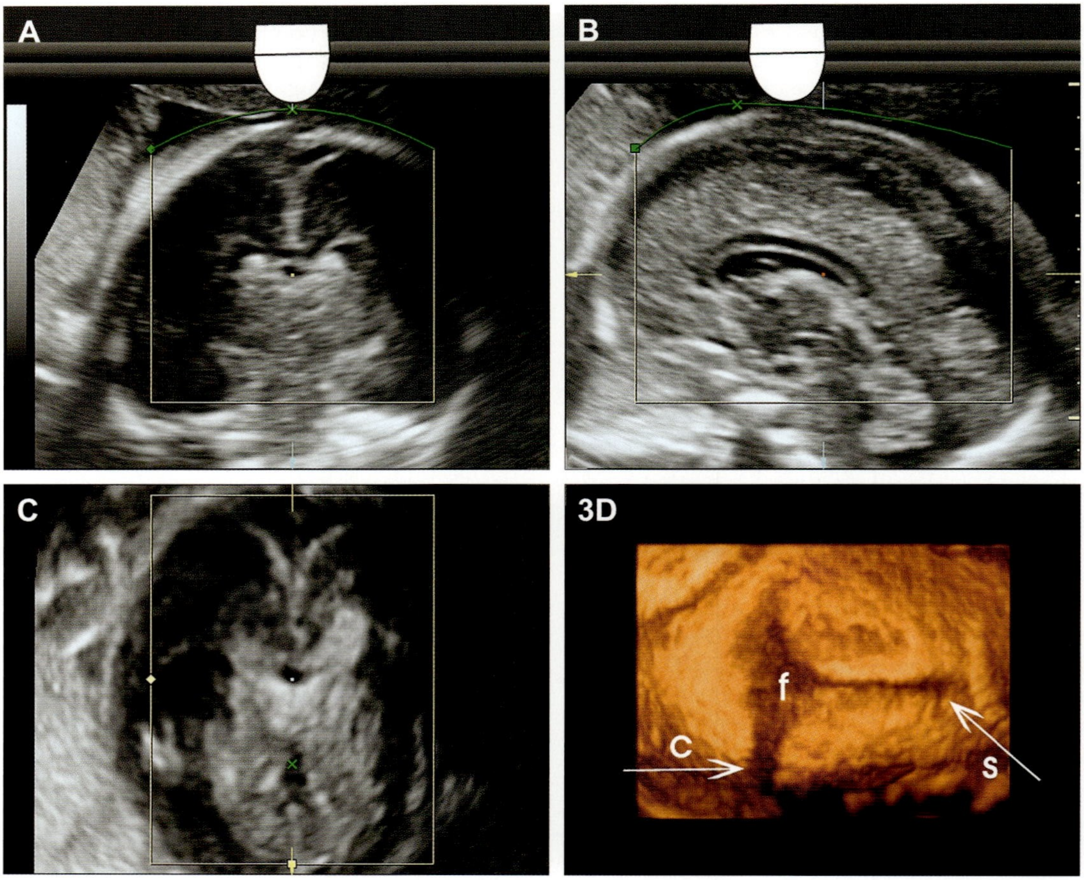

Fig. 2. Multiplanar image of the fetal brain acquired transabdominally. Note that the beam of the probe is directed toward the anterior fontanelle (Boxes A and B). Box 3D demonstrates a surface rendering of the fetal scalp at the area to which the probe is directed. Even with a transabdominal approach, a good image can be achieved by directing the beam through the anterior fontanelle (f). The sagittal (s) and coronal (c) are also displayed (Box 3D).

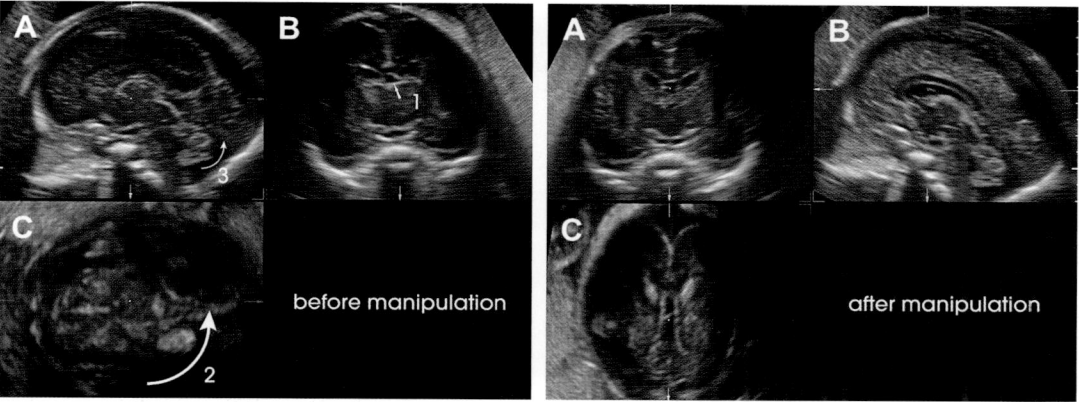

Fig. 3. The multiplanar mode panel on the left side (before manipulation) displays the initial image of the acquired brain volume after the image was enlarged to fit the whole screen. Several steps were taken manipulating the volume to obtain the desired orientation. (1) The marker dot in Box B was moved to the center of the fetal brain (cavum septi pellucidi, in this case) (*arrow*). (2) The axial image in Box C was rotated 90° on the z-plane to place the fetal head in the axial plane, with the forehead pointing down (*large curved arrow*). (3) At this point, the mid-coronal position will be displayed in Box A, and only slight rotations may be required to fine-tune it in the perfect orientation (*small curved arrow*). The multiplanar display on the right side (after manipulation) demonstrates the same volume in the correct orientation after completing the above three steps. The authors prefer to display the images in the multiplanar mode, with the coronal plane in perfect alignment in Box A, in the median plane with the fetus "looking" to the left in Box B, and the axial plane with the fetal forehead pointing downwards in Box C.

in the multiplanar panel on the right side of **Fig. 3** (after manipulation).

Box A should now display a coronal section of the brain. At the same time, on the sagittal image in Box B, the moving vertical line displays the level at which the picture in Box A is seen (see **Fig. 3**).

By moving the marker dot horizontally from side to side on the coronal plane (Box A), successive sagittal sections from side-to-side (temporal-to-temporal) can be imaged in Box B following the planes of the sections in the coronal image. These successive sagittal images are displayed in **Fig. 4** by using the Tomographic ultrasound imaging (TUI) mode.

Finally, moving the marker dot up and down on the coronal plane (Box A), successive horizontal (axial) views of the brain from the base of the skull to the "top-of-the-head" can be imaged on Box C. These successive axial planes are displayed in **Fig. 5** using the TUI display mode.

Manipulating the Volume to Obtain Diagnostic Planes

Manipulating the 3D-ultrasound volume in the multiplanar mode as described earlier enables a relatively easy reconstruction of several diagnostic planes. However, before starting to navigate in the acquired volume, one has to acknowledge that the number of possibilities is virtually endless. One should remember that the display protocol of different manufacturers may be different. A repetitive manipulation of a volume is a good training tool to master the display technique of each specific brand. In the authors' experience, a complete neuroscan can be efficiently performed using five to seven continuous coronal sections, three sagittal sections (including the median and two parasagittal sections), and three axial sections. Recently, the International Society of Ultrasound in Obstetrics and Gynecology (ISUOG) published guidelines recommending the necessary planes to be used in dedicated neurosonography, in addition to the axial planes that are routinely performed. They included four coronal planes—the transfrontal, transcaudate, transthalamic and transcerebellar—as well as three sagittal planes: median and two parasagittal.[6] These recommendations did not include a 3D-brain scan; however, all these recommended planes can be visualized in few minutes after the perfect orientation of a good quality volume is obtained in the three orthogonal planes.

The median plane

The median plane is probably the most important plane, as it enables evaluation of several important midline brain structures. The median plane of the fetal brain can be used to assess the corpus callosum, the cavum septi pellucidi,

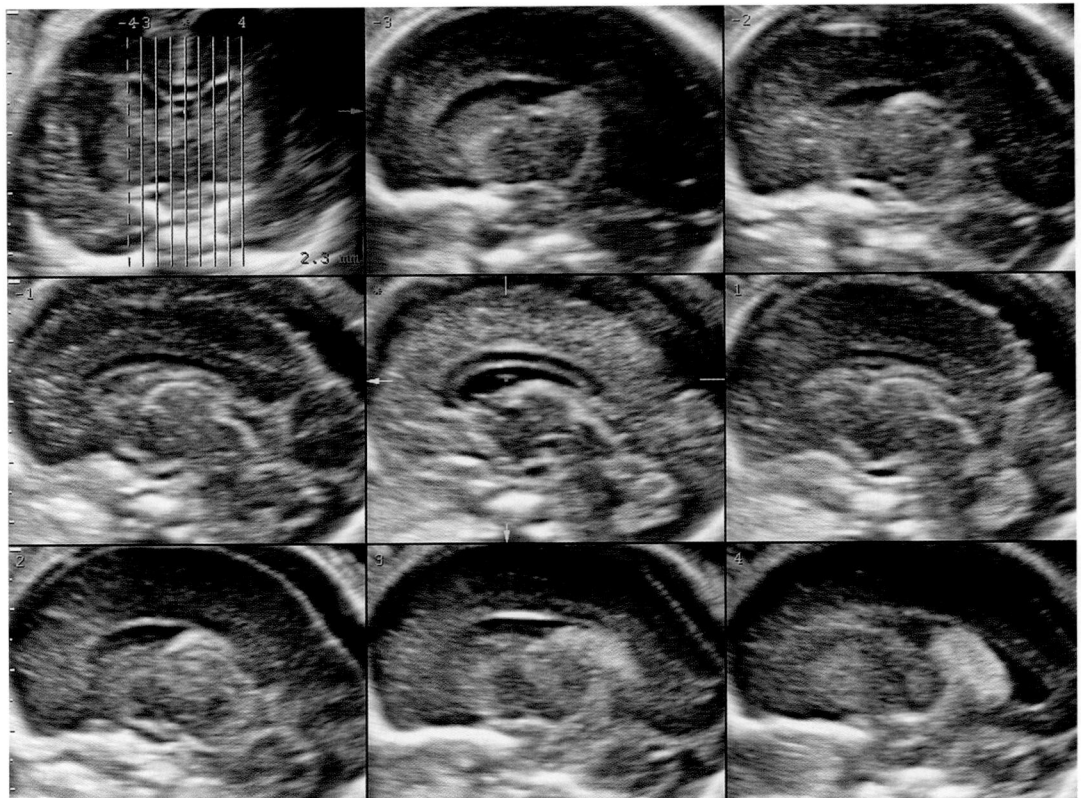

Fig. 4. Tomographic display mode demonstrating multiple successive sagittal views of the fetal brain. These successive sections can also be seen in the multiplanar mode Box B, when the marker dot (*red dot*) on the coronal view in Box A is moved horizontally from side to side on the initial orthogonal plane.

the cavum vergae, the head of the caudate nucleus, the tela choroidea, the quadrigeminal plate, the quadrigeminal cistern, the cavum veli interpositi, the brain stem, the pons, the third and fourth ventricles, the cerebellar vermis, the cisterna magna, and the nuchal fold. **Fig. 6** demonstrates a perfect median plane that was obtained by 3D manipulation. This image is displayed side by side with an identical image that has several midline anatomic structures marked with arrows. In the "perfect" median plane, one should not see the thalami. However, because any ultrasound plane has a third plane (thin as it may be), it is possible to see slices of the thalami that most of the time are so close to each other that they touch. Depending on the fetal position, the acquisition of the median plane may be impossible with 2D-transabdominal ultrasound and require special expertise in transvaginal-transfontanelle scanning, as well as prolonged examination time. Obtaining the median plane by manipulation of 3D-ultrasound volume can be easily obtained by aligning all three planes according to the previously described protocol and placing the marker dot in the center of the coronal plane.

The authors have previously demonstrated that 3D reconstruction is useful in evaluating the integrity of the corpus callosum and in diagnosing complete or partial agenesis, as well as evaluating the entire lateral ventricles.[7] Several other studies focused on the median plane as a useful method for brain anomaly detection.[8–10] The authors have found the tomographic display mode to be extremely informative in the examination of the fetal brain by displaying consecutive parasagittal planes with the midsagittal plane.

The three-horn view: parasagittal

Several methods of evaluating the ventricular system have been described, with the standard measurement of the atrium (or body) of the lateral ventricle in the axial plane being the most common, as demonstrated in **Fig. 7**.[2–4,9,11–13] When ventriculomegaly occurs, the posterior horn is the first to change in size and shape and the

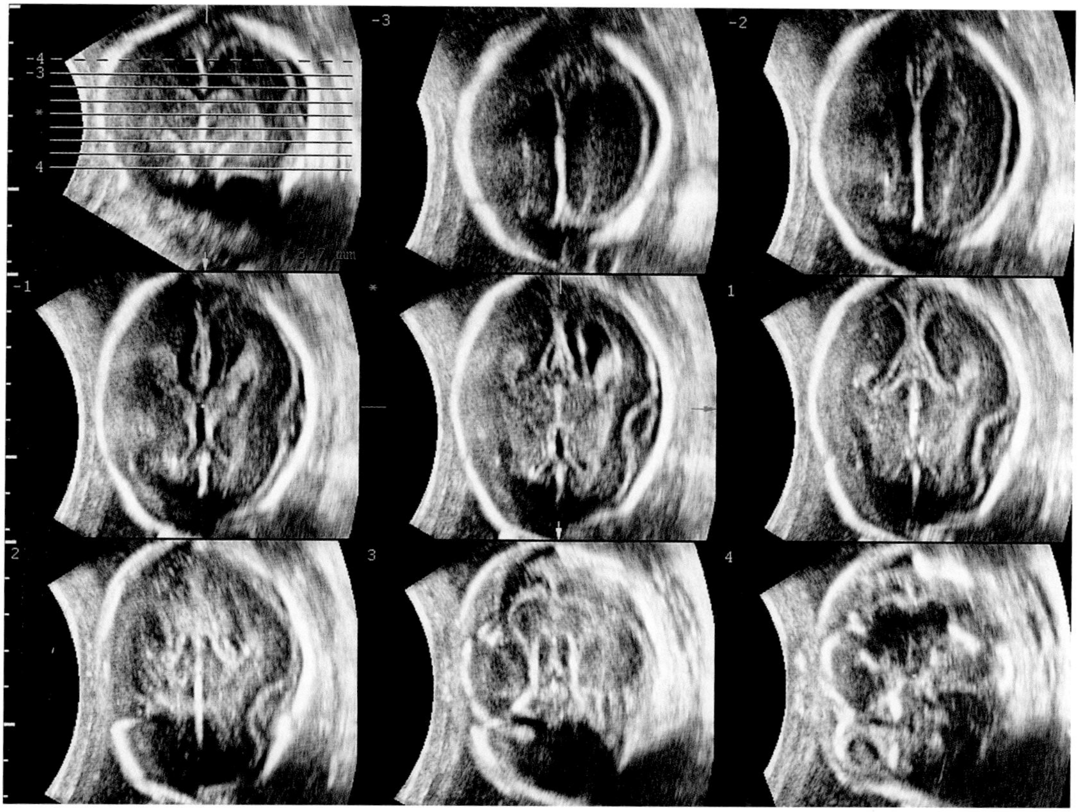

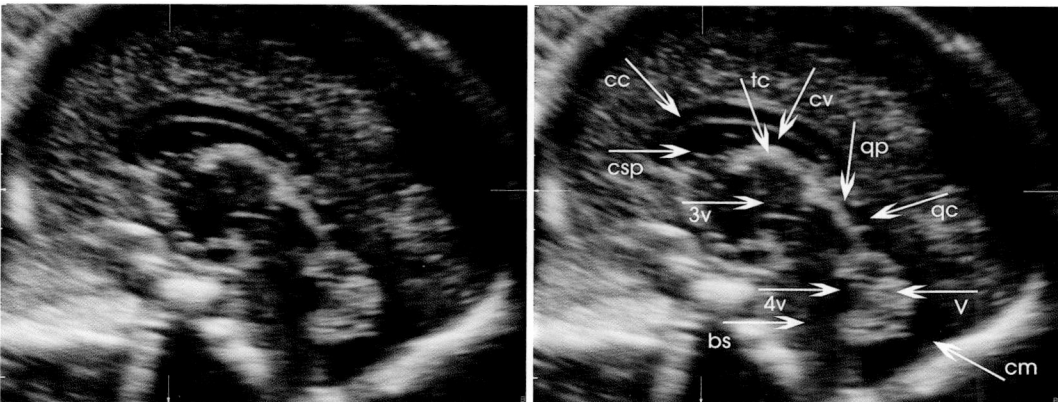

Fig. 5. Tomographic display mode, demonstrating multiple successive axial views of the fetal brain. These successive sections can also be seen in Box C of the multiplanar display mode by moving the marker dot in the coronal plane in Box A up and down on the initial orthogonal plane.

Fig. 6. These identical images of the "perfect" median plane obtained from a multiplanar display mode demonstrate the anatomic location of several midline brain structures. The arrows point to the corpus callosum (cc), cavum septi pellucidi (csp), tela choroidea (tc), cavum vergae (cv), quadrigeminal plate (qp), quadrigeminal cistern (qc), third ventricle (3v), fourth ventricle (4v), brain stem (bs), cerebellar vermis (V), and the cisterna magna (cm).

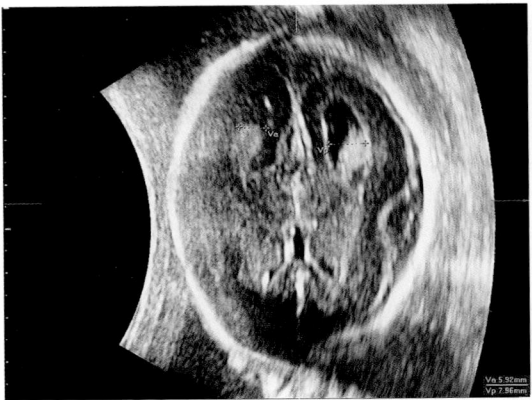

Fig. 7. Standard axial plane taken at the level of the lateral ventricles and cavum septi pellucidi, demonstrating measurements of the lateral ventricles. Note that the proximal ventricle (*left*) is not clearly seen because of "noise" and reverberations that decrease the quality of the image. Va, left lateral ventricle; Vp, right lateral ventricle.

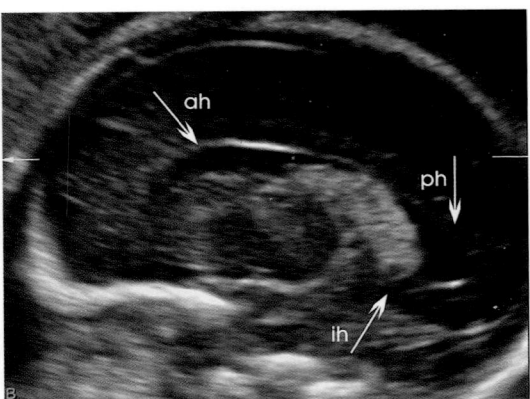

Fig. 8. The three-horn view in this image enables the evaluation of all three components of the lateral ventricles. The arrows point to the anterior horn (ah), posterior horn (ph), and inferior horn (ih).

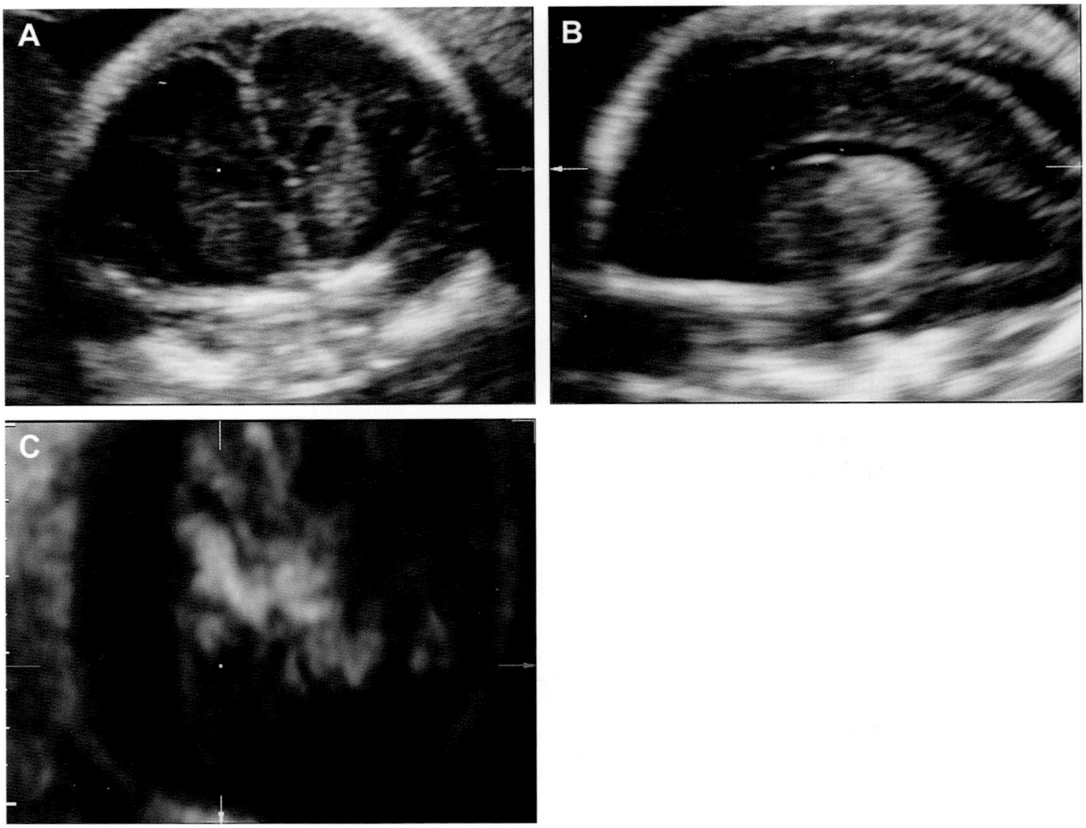

Fig. 9. Multiplanar mode demonstrating the specific alignment of the three orthogonal planes necessary to obtain the 3HV. The marker dot is placed in the left anterior horn and the coronal plane (Box A) is tilted slightly to the left on the *z*-axis. The axial plane (Box C) is also tilted slightly to the left on the *z*-axis. The sagittal plane in Box B than displays the 3HV.

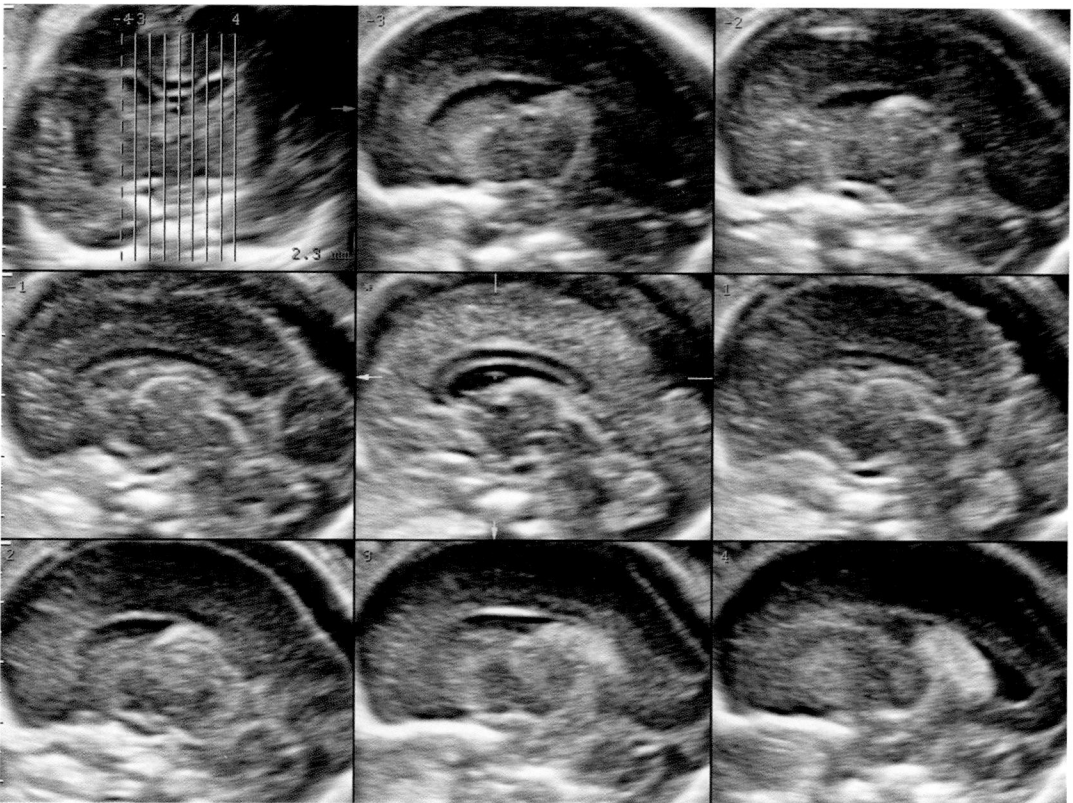

Fig. 10. Tomographic display mode of multiple sagittal views including the median plane (*middle*) and the parasagittal views, enabling evaluation of both lateral ventricles.

easiest to evaluate on the axial plane. The anterior horn is the last portion of the lateral ventricle to dilate.[14,15] The inferior horn is either barely visible or not visible earlier in pregnancy. The parasagittal plane, which we have termed the "three-horn view" (3HV), enables all three horns of the lateral ventricle to be displayed on one image (**Fig. 8**). The ventricular system is positioned obliquely within the brain, with the anterior horns closer to each other than the distance between the posterior horns. Additionally, the distance between the inferior horns is even larger. Using 3D technique to obtain this view is both simple and rapid, by tilting the volume on the coronal plane using the y- and z-axis. **Fig. 9** displays a multiplanar mode that demonstrates the necessary tilting in the coronal plane (Box A), and the axial plane (Box C) to obtain the 3HV. An easy way to evaluate the lateral ventricles is by multiple, successive sagittal slices using the TUI mode (**Fig. 10**).

The three horns should be considered abnormal in several situations:[11]

> If the anterior horn height is larger than 8.7 mm at 14 weeks and 6.9 mm at 40 weeks (represent the 95th percentile for these measurements);
> If the posterior horn height is larger than 11 mm at 14 weeks and 14 mm at 39 weeks (represent the 95th percentile for these measurements);
> If the posterior horn measurement from the posterior tip of the thalamus to the posterior tip of the horn is larger than 2.6 mm at 14 weeks to 3.4 mm at 40 weeks (represent the 95th percentile for these measurements);
> If the inferior horn is obvious to any degree.

The 3HV provides an objective measure evaluating both the severity of the ventricular dilatation and the progression of the pathology with successive measurements that are facilitated in this plane. Another use of the 3HV is the recognition of colpocephaly, a pathologic and persistent dilatation of the posterior horn, which has been associated with agenesis of the corpus callosum and other syndromes affecting the midbrain, such as obstruction of the aqueduct.[16] Some believe that not all cases of colpocephaly are a result of pressure-related anomalies, but may be a result

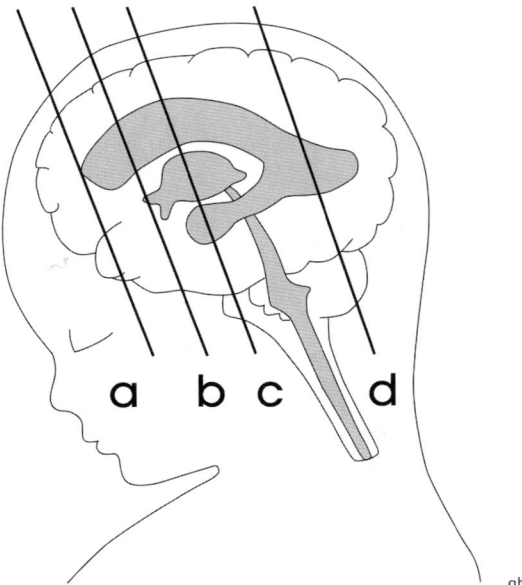

Fig. 11. Fetal head in the sagittal position, demonstrating the anatomic position of the successive coronal planes that are recommended by the ISUOG during the fetal neuroscan. Transfrontal plane (a), transcaudate (b), transthalamic (c), and transcerebellar (d).

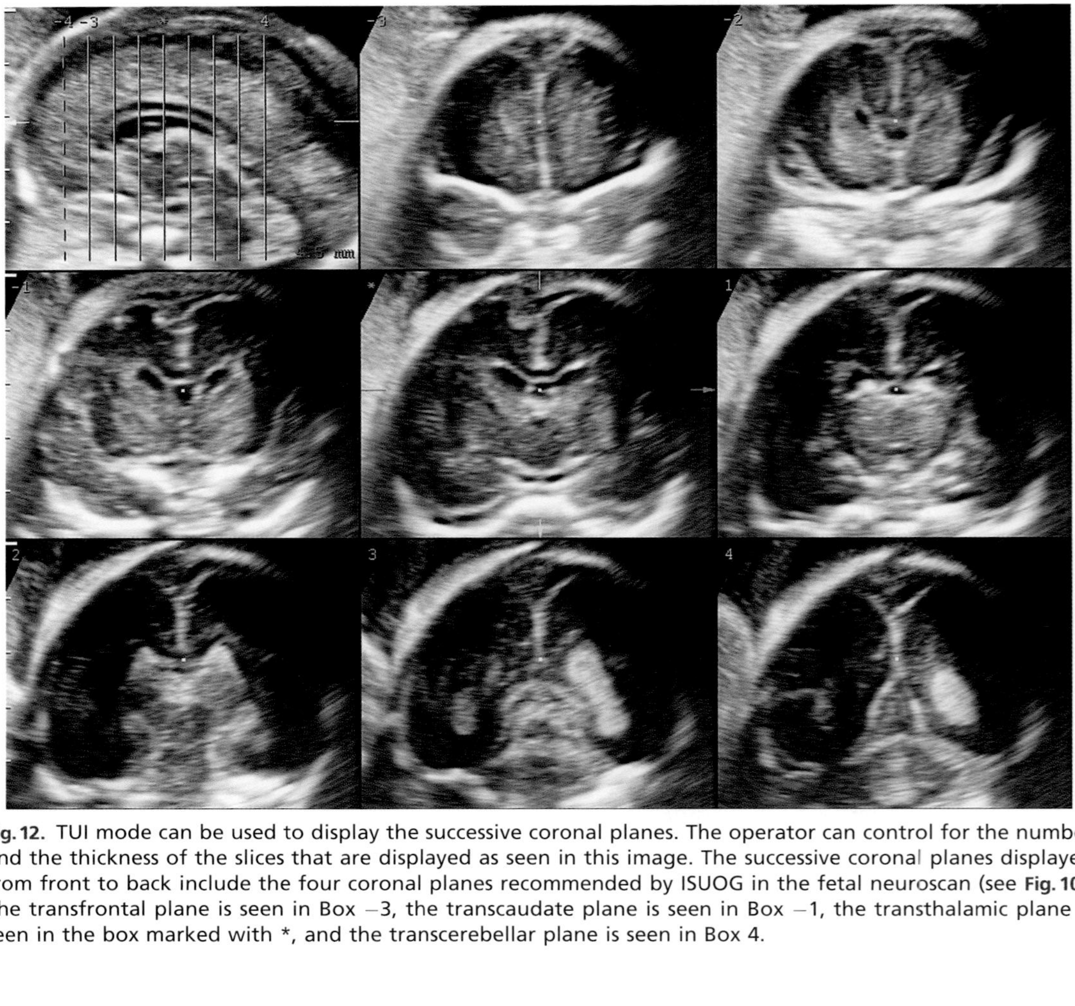

Fig. 12. TUI mode can be used to display the successive coronal planes. The operator can control for the number and the thickness of the slices that are displayed as seen in this image. The successive coronal planes displayed from front to back include the four coronal planes recommended by ISUOG in the fetal neuroscan (see **Fig. 10**). The transfrontal plane is seen in Box −3, the transcaudate plane is seen in Box −1, the transthalamic plane is seen in the box marked with *, and the transcerebellar plane is seen in Box 4.

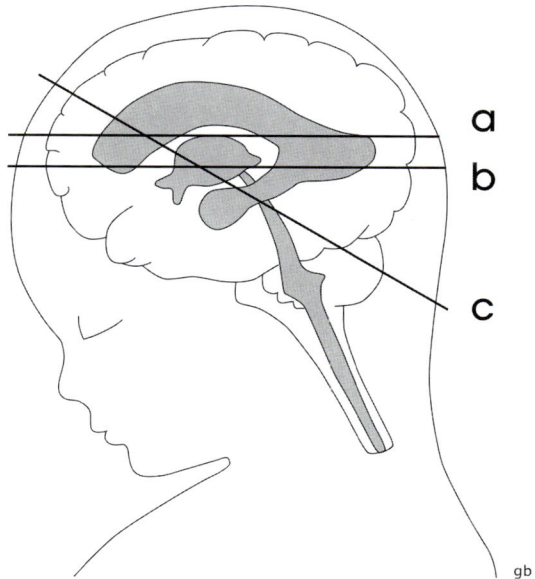

Fig. 13. This diagram of a fetal head in the sagittal position illustrates the correct anatomic position of the three axial planes: the transventricular (a), transthalamic (b), and transcerebellar (c).

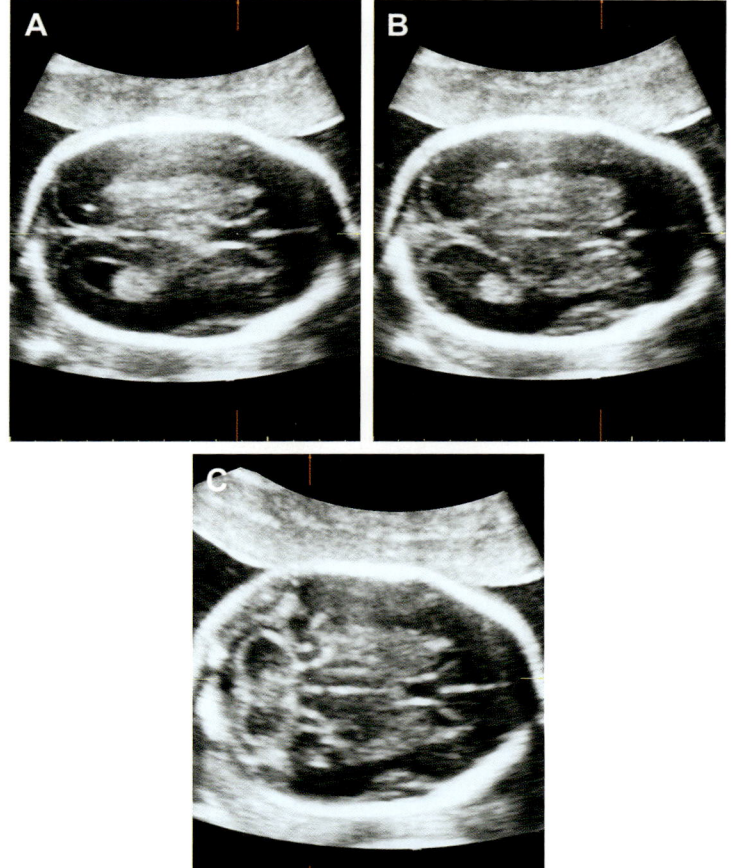

Fig. 14. Examples of 3D ultrasound reconstructions of the commonly used axial planes: transventricular (*A*), transthalamic (*B*), and transcerebellar (*C*).

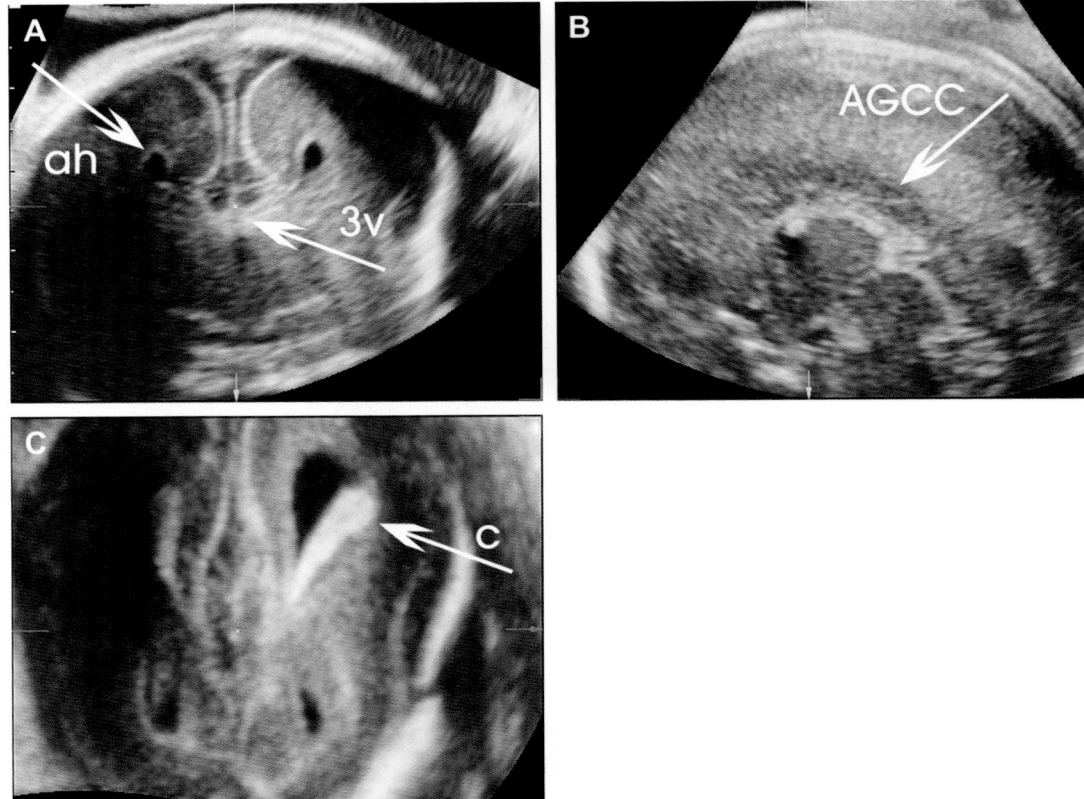

Fig. 15. Multiplanar display of a fetus with agenesis of the corpus callosum. The diagnosis can be made based upon its direct signs on the "perfect median" plane in Box B, demonstrating the absence of the corpus callosum (*arrow* AGCC), and absence of the cavum septi pellucidi (Box B). The coronal image in Box A demonstrates the widely spaced anterior horns (ah) showing the classic "Viking's helmet sign," and the interhemispheric fissure connecting all the way to the upward displaced third ventricle (3v). The axial image in Box C demonstrates the parallel lateral ventricles and the colpocephaly (c), which are characteristic to this anomaly.

of an error in morphogenesis.[17] Heinz and colleagues[18] were able to distinguish between obstructive and atrophic dilatation of the lateral ventricles in 92 infants and children using CT. Obstructive dilatations showed a much larger measurement of the inferior and anterior horns than the posterior horn. However, in cases of atrophic dilatation, colpocephaly was more prominent. It only seems logical to employ the 3HV in differentiating the above-mentioned obstructive and atrophic entities based on the ventricular horn dilatation.

Another use of the 3HV is to compare the size and shape of the left lateral ventricle to the right lateral ventricles in the same fetus. Although minimal asymmetry between the lateral ventricles may exist,[12,18,19] precise measurements of the size of the left and right lateral ventricles in cases of lateral ventricular asymmetry contributed to an objective identification of pathologic unilateral dilatation.[20]

Coronal plane

Using the transvaginal-transfontanelle approach, diagnostic views of the fetal brain in the coronal plane can be obtained. Navigating through the brain using the multiplanar display modality, the marker dot is moved on the axial plane in Box C from the front of the head to the back of the head along the midline, or on the B plane from anterior to posterior. By doing so, continuous sections of the fetal brain in the coronal plane in Box A are obtained. The authors usually observe five to seven of these successive coronal planes, including the ones recommended by ISUOG: that is, the transfrontal, transcaudate, transthalamic and transcerebellar planes (**Fig. 11**).[6] These planes can be seen in the TUI display in **Fig. 12**. The transfrontal plane demonstrates the uninterrupted interhemispheric fissure in the midline, with the anterior horns in the sides. The orbits and the sphenoidal bone may be seen as well.

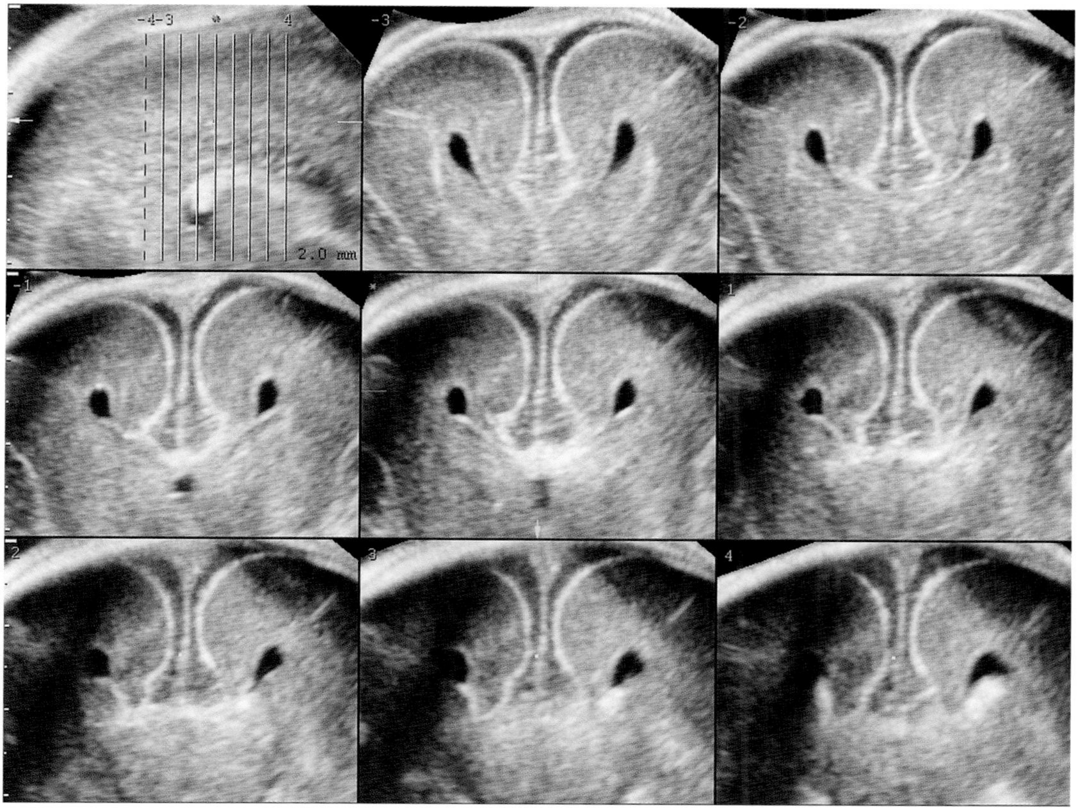

Fig. 16. Tomographic display mode demonstrating successive coronal views of the same fetus with AGCC. The absence of the corpus can be diagnosed based on the "Viking's helmet sign" and the upward displacement of the third ventricle that connects with the interhemispheric fissure. This modality is helpful in differentiating partial from total agenesis of the corpus callosum.

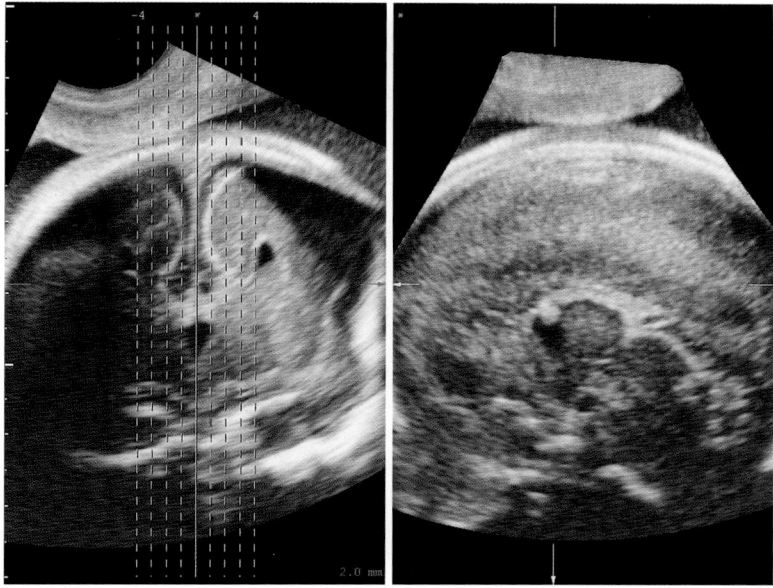

Fig. 17. Side-by-side display of the tomographic display mode may be used to enhance the typical findings of AGCC in these coronal and median planes.

The transcaudate plane is taken at the level of the caudate nuclei, with the interhemispheric fissure interrupted by the genu of the corpus callosum. The cavum septum pellucidi can be seen under the corpus callosum and the lateral ventricles in each side.

The transthalamic plane is taken at the level of thalami and can be used to evaluate its integrity.

The transcerebellar plane is frequently used to evaluate the posterior fossa, demonstrating the occipital horns of the lateral ventricles, interhemispheric fissure, and the cerebellum.

Axial planes

Similarly to the 2D basic fetal brain evaluation, the axial planes that are obtained during the 3D neuroscan are the transventricular plane, the transcerebellar plane (which is taken in a lower level with a posterior tilt), and the intermediate transthalamic biparietal diameter plane (**Figs. 13** and **14**). These planes provide information regarding various brain structures, depending on the level in which it crosses the brain. Among these structures are the fetal scull, falx cerebri, gyri and sulci, thalami, cavum septi pellucidi, the posterior horn of the lateral ventricles, the choroid plexus, the cerebellum, cisterna magna, and nuchal fold. The evaluation of these planes using a 3D technique may be facilitated by the simultaneous observation of the sagittal plane and the precise angle in which the axial is crossing it to achieve the desired planes. Of note, better quality of the axial plane is achieved when the volume is acquired in this plane. In cases in which the axial plane is reconstructed, the quality will be inferior to the one obtained by the 2D technique.

DETECTION OF FETAL NEUROPATHOLOGY BY 3D ULTRASOUND

This section presents several examples of how the authors use 3D-ultrasound in the diagnosis and work-up of several brain anomalies.

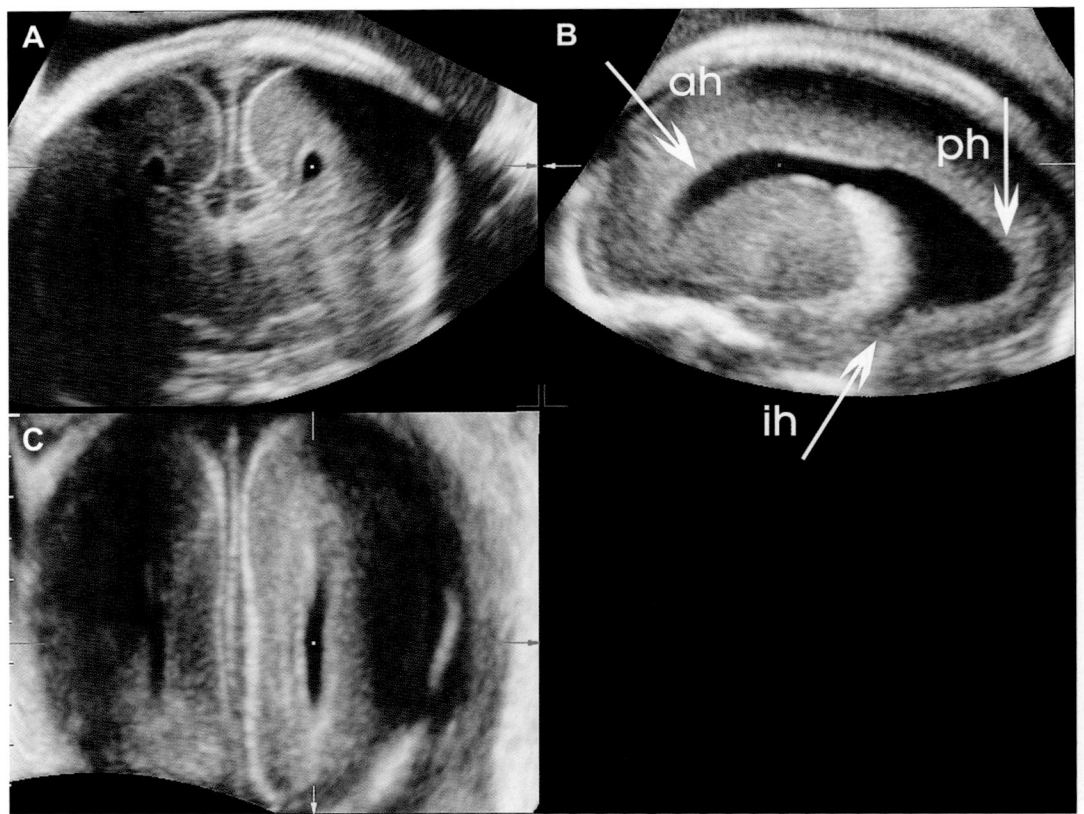

Fig. 18. Multiplanar display focusing on the ventricular system. The coronal plane in Box A demonstrates the widely spaced anterior horns (Viking's helmet sign). The axial plane in Box C displays the abnormally parallel lateral ventricles. The 3HV is obtained in Box B, demonstrating the abnormally dilated lateral ventricle. The arrows mark the anterior horn (ah), posterior horn (ph), and inferior horn (ih) that comprise the lateral ventricle.

Agenesis of the Corpus Callosum

The corpus callosum starts to form at around 12 weeks of gestation and completes its anterior-to-posterior development at around 20 to 22 postmenstrual weeks. Failure of axons to cross the midline and form the corpus callosum results in partial or total agenesis of the corpus callosum (AGCC) (absence of the entire corpus callosum or partial development of its anterior part only). In spite of the fact that this diagnosis can be made based upon axial and coronal sections revealing the indirect signs of the malformation, the direct diagnosis of the absence of the corpus callosum can only be obtained by the median plane. The median plane is obtained almost exclusively by the transvaginal scanning approach, provided the fetus is in vertex presentation. The authors' experience in evaluating patients referred for second-opinion for hydrocephaly or ventriculomegaly has led to the belief that many cases of AGCC are often misdiagnosed. This might be because of the lack of expertise necessary to obtain the diagnostic median plane performing a transvaginal neuroscan. As described earlier, the manipulation of the 3D volume is extremely useful in detecting midline structures and, hence, the application of this modality in abnormalities of the corpus callosum is clinically helpful and may improve the detection of this anomaly.

The median plane facilitates the inspection of the anatomic site of the corpus callosum, the cavum septi pellucidi, and the pericallosal artery enabling the diagnosis of AGCC. Additional indirect findings

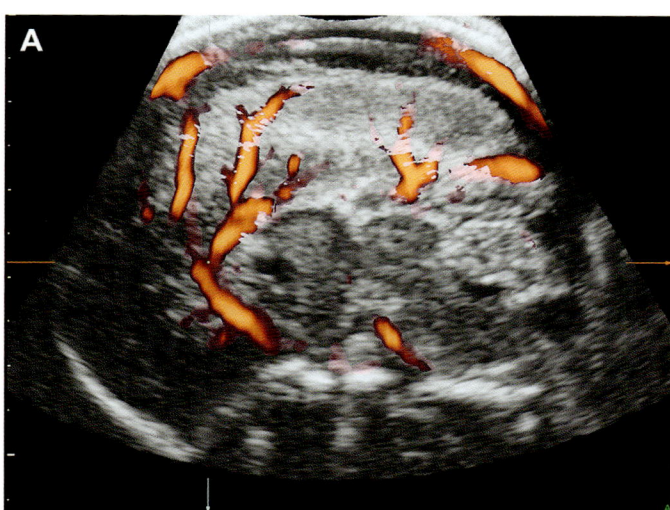

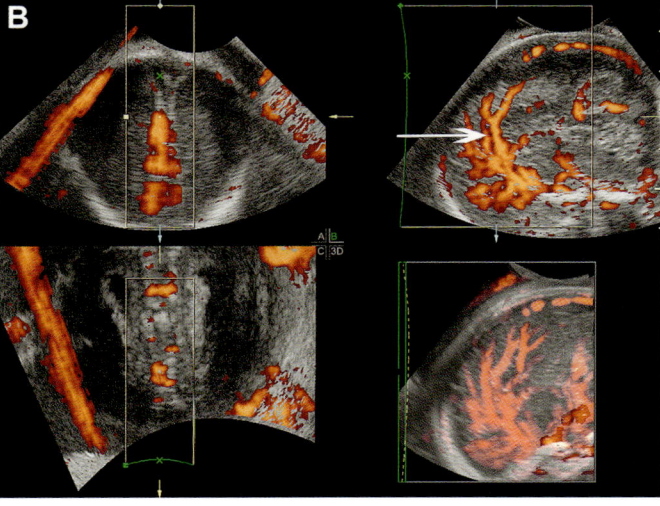

Fig. 19. Angiographic demonstrations of brain vessels in AGCC. (*A*) Three-dimesional power Doppler angiography-acquired median plane demonstrating the anterior cerebral artery and the absence of the pericallosal artery branch. (*B*) Three-dimesional power Doppler angiography multiplanar display mode demonstrating the anterior cerebral artery (*arrow*) and the absence of the pericallosal artery. The "thick slice" technique was used to obtain a 3D rendering of the brain vasculature (Box 3D) displaying the anterior cerebral artery and the absence of the pericallosal artery.

associated with this anomaly may be seen on different diagnostic planes and include:

- Teardrop-shaped, parallel lateral ventricles seen on the axial section;
- Colpocephaly: a dilated posterior horn can be seen on the axial and 3HVs;
- "Sunburst sign": radial gyri and sulci on median surface (seen only after 26 to 28 weeks when gyri/sulci are normally visible) on the median section;
- "Viking's helmet sign": widely separated, vertically oriented lateral ventricles seen on the anterior coronal sections;
- Upward displacement of the third ventricle connecting with the interhemispheric fissure on the coronal section.

Figs. 15 to **18** demonstrate a case of AGCC in which simple manipulation of the volume of the brain enabled visualization of both the direct and indirect signs, leading to a clear diagnosis within few minutes. As described earlier, the appropriate volume orientation is obtained using the multiplanar mode to achieve the three orthogonal planes perfectly placed in the midline position. **Fig. 15** demonstrates a multiplanar mode with the median plane in Box B, providing direct sonographic evidence of the absence of the corpus callosum (*arrow*, AGCC) and the absence of the cavum septi pellucidi. The image in the mid-coronal plane in Box A clearly demonstrates the widely displaced and upward pointing anterior horns (*arrow*, ah) of the lateral ventricles (Viking's helmet sign), and the elevation of the third ventricle (*arrow*, 3v), which is contiguous with the interhemispheric fissure. These findings can be further enhanced using the tomographic display mode to obtain successive coronal sections, which were extremely helpful in providing MR imaging-like diagnostic images (**Figs. 16** and **17**). Scrolling up and down through the axial image in Box C of the multiplanar display mode (see **Fig. 15**), the authors could appreciate the characteristic teardrop-shaped and parallel lateral ventricles with dilated posterior horns, colpocephaly (*arrow*, c). This finding can be further enhanced by obtaining the 3HV (**Fig. 18**), in which the entire dilated lateral ventricle is evident with the overly dilated posterior horn known as colpocephaly (Box B).

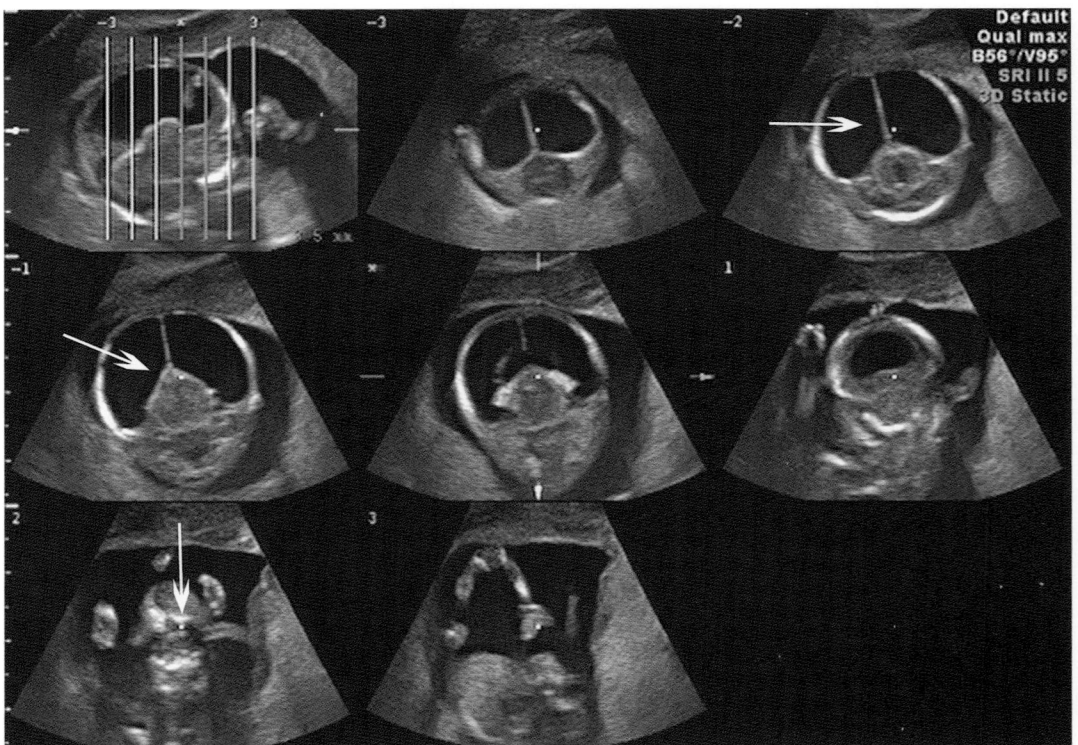

Fig. 20. Tomographic display mode showing multiple successive coronal views in a fetus with semi-lobar holoprosencephaly diagnosed at 12 postmenstrual weeks. The arrows point to the incomplete falx (Box −2) that is seen on the posterior portion of the brain but not on the anterior portion (Box 1), and to the fused thalami (Box −1). The typical hypotelorism can be seen in the anterior coronal view in Box 2 (*arrow*).

The use of 3D color Doppler is very helpful in diagnosing AGCC and sometimes is the only direct clue in cases with a challenging scan. **Fig. 19** demonstrates 3D volumes that were acquired with the power Doppler turned on, while focusing on the area of the corpus callosum in two different cases of AGCC. Clearly, in both images, only the anterior cerebellar artery is detected and the pericallosal artery was not seen branching from it, confirming the diagnosis of AGCC in these cases at 20 and 22 postmenstrual weeks, respectively. The power Doppler technique is especially important in cases of partial agenesis of the corpus callosum detecting the anterior portion (but not the entire) pericallosal artery branching off of the anterior cerebral artery. Additionally, a small anterior portion of the genu corporis callosi, as well as a small cavum septi pellucidi, may be seen in such cases.

Using the 3D neuroscan to identify this anomaly, as well as other anomalies, it is important to obtain a perfect median plane. Correlation with other orthogonal planes is required to ensure that the section is properly oriented and that the diagnostic image is indeed in the true median plane.

Holoprosencephaly

Holoprosencephaly is associated with an incidense of 1 per 1,600 births, but is detected more frequently when earlier sonograms are performed. The sonographic detection of the frequent forms, Alobar and Semilobar types, is relatively straight forward. Absence of the interhemispheric fissure (total or partial), nondisjunction of the thalami, absence of the corpus callosum and cavum septi pellucidi, and various facial anomalies (cyclops, proboscis, median clefts, and other anomalies) are the most frequent sonographic features. The authors' experience performing 3D neuroscan enabled accurate diagnosis of this complex syndrome in several cases during the first trimester. The authors demonstrate a case of a fetus with semi-lobar holoprosencephaly diagnosed at 12 postmenstrual weeks. The manipulation of the brain volume in this case was extremely helpful in displaying the images in a diagnostic fashion. **Fig. 20** is a TUI of multiple coronal sections demonstrating the falx (*arrow* in Box −2), which is not detected in the anterior section of the brain (Box 1), revealing the connection of the two ventricles at the level of the anterior horns. The fused thalami

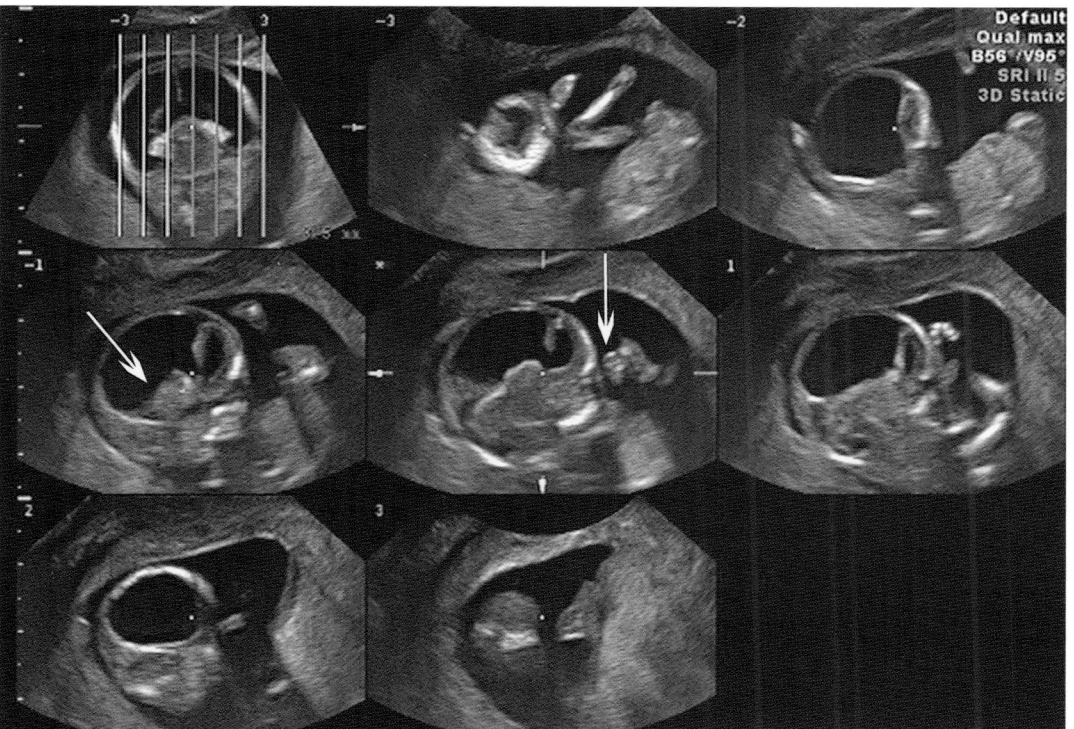

Fig. 21. Tomographic display mode showing multiple successive sagittal views in this fetus with semi-lobar holoprosencephaly. The arrows point to the fused thalami (Box −1), and to the abnormal proboscis (Box marked with *). The massive hydrocephaly is very obvious.

is detected in Box −1 (*arrow*). The typical hypotelorism can be also appreciated in the facial coronal view in Box 2 (see marker dot in Box 2). The sagittal TUI in **Fig. 21** demonstrate the fused thalami (*arrow*, Box −1), and the facial proboscis (*arrow* in Box *). **Fig. 22** is a multiplanar mode of the same case demonstrating the anomaly in the three orthogonal planes. An inversion mode is displayed in Box 3D, demonstrating the entire ventricular system. The massive hydrocephaly can be appreviated, as well as the two hemispheres that are partially separated by the falx (*arrow*) in the opsterior part, whereas the anterior part of the ventricles is connected (*double arrow*). An example of inversion mode and multiplanar display in a case of alobar holoprosencephaly is shown in **Fig. 23**.

The lobar type has a more subtle sonographic features, which are clustered around the corpus callosum, cavum septi pellucidi, and the third ventricle. The presence of a box-shaped cavity in the midbrain below the corpus callosum, without the two lateral walls of the septum pellucidum, suggests the presence of either lobar holoprosencephaly or septo-optic dysplasia. The final diagnosis between the two may not be made until after birth.

Cephalocele

This anomaly is characterized by herniation of intracranial structures through a skull defect. It was reported to occur in approximately 1 to 3 out of every 10,000 live births. The most common form of cephalocele is the encephalocele that consists of both brain and meninges herniating through the skull. Meningocele, however, is a less-severe defect in which only the meninges are herniating through the skull defect to the para-cranial mass. There is large variation in the location and extent of this anomaly, which is usually associated with the location of the scull sutures. About 80% of all cases among the white population in both Europe and North America are localized in the occipital region, with cases occurring in the temporal and

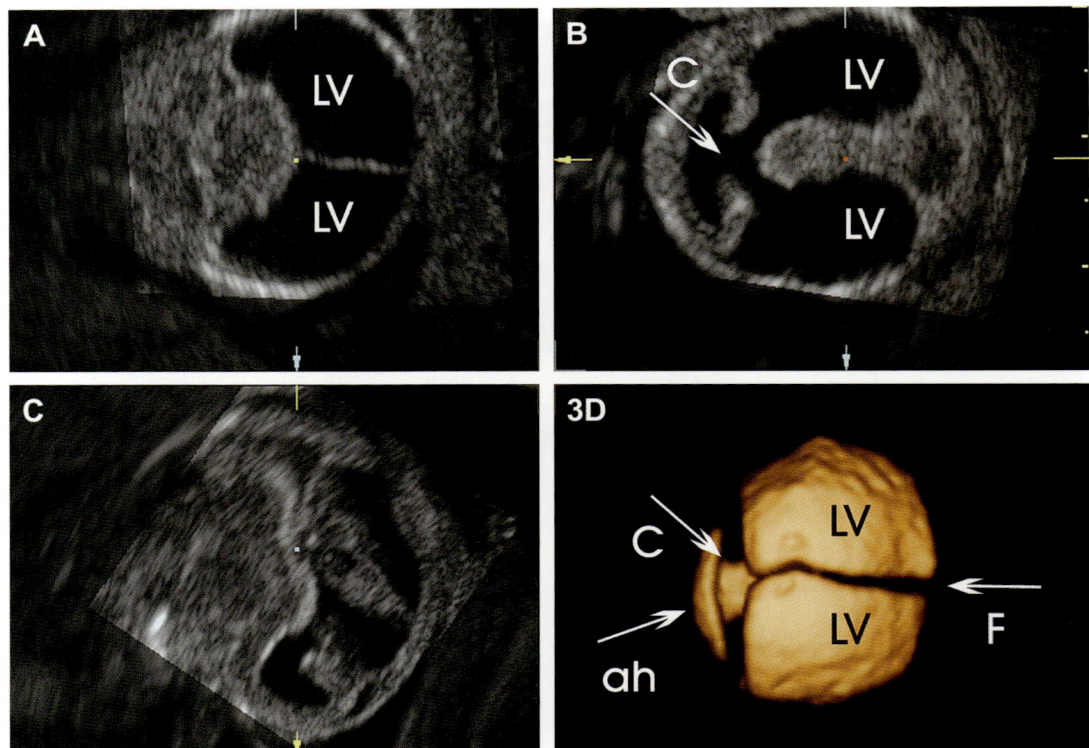

Fig. 22. Multiplanar mode of the same fetus with semi-lobar holoprosencephaly. The falx and fused thalami are seen in Box A. The incomplete falx is seen in Box B (see *marker dot*) and the two lateral ventricles (LV) are seen with a clear communication (*arrow*, C) making the diagnosis of semi-lobar holoprosencephaly. Inversion mode rendering is demonstrated in Box 3D identifying the two dilated ventricles (LV) with their communication (*arrow*, C) at the level of the anterior horns (ah). The black line between the two ventricles (*arrow*, F) represents the posterior segment of the falx.

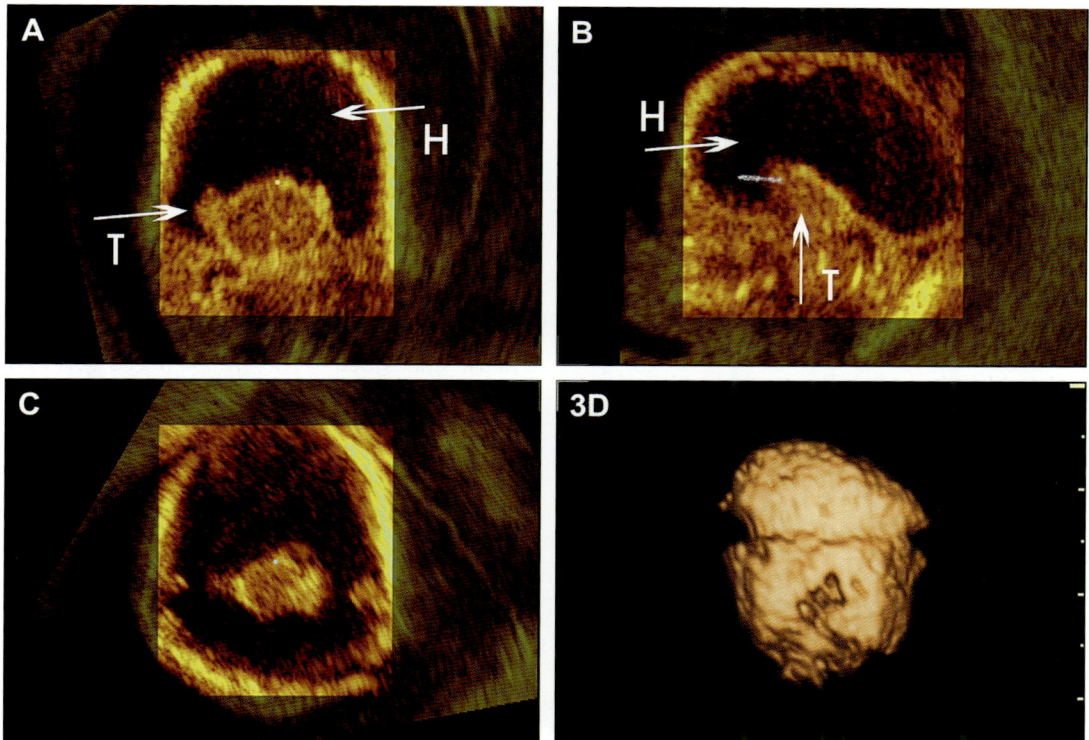

Fig. 23. Multiplanar view of a case of alobar holoprosencephaly. The orthogonal planes display the fused thalami (*arrow*, T) and the markedly dilated and completely fused ventricles that are characteristic of holoprosencephaly (*arrow*, H). No falx is present, making the diagnosis consistent with the alobar form. The inversion mode is seen in Box 3D, demonstrating a superior view of the large fluid-filled space representing the fused dilated ventricles.

frontal region less frequently. In contrast, among the Southeast Asian population, the most common location is the fronto-ethmoidal region. Parietal cephaloceles are the least common and are mostly associated with significant underlying brain anomalies. Cephalocele should be suspected when a para-cranial mass is detected on ultrasound. In the authors' experience, the additive value of 3D ultrasound in the diagnosis of these anomalies lies mainly in the ability to navigate with the marker dot through the skull defect and demonstrate the connection of the brain to the adjacent cystic structure. In few difficult cases, where this connection was not detected by fetal brain MR imaging, the authors were able to detect the specific site of the communication using this technique (**Fig. 24**). In this case, the authors have also used power Doppler angiography to demonstrate blood vessel crossing the cranial defect, confirming the diagnosis of occipital meningyocele, as can be seen in **Figs. 25** and **26**.

Arachnoid Cysts

Arachnoid cyst is a collection of cerebrospinal fluid within layers of arachnoid that is not connected with the ventricular system. It is a benign space-occupying lesion, the significance of which is dependent on its location and the extent of compression on the surrounding structures. It may be located in various parts of the brain, such as in its surface, between the lobes, and even in the depth of the brain originating at various sites. It is more commonly detected on the left side of the brain. In 5% to 10% of cases, the cyst may be located in the posterior fossa, resulting in upward displacement of the tentorium and vermis. However, in this case the anatomy of the cerebellum and the fourth ventricle remains normal, differentiating it from other posterior-fossa anomalies, such as the Dandy Walker malformation. Many cysts remain stable in size and do not compress vital brain structures. Occasionally, large arachnoid cysts

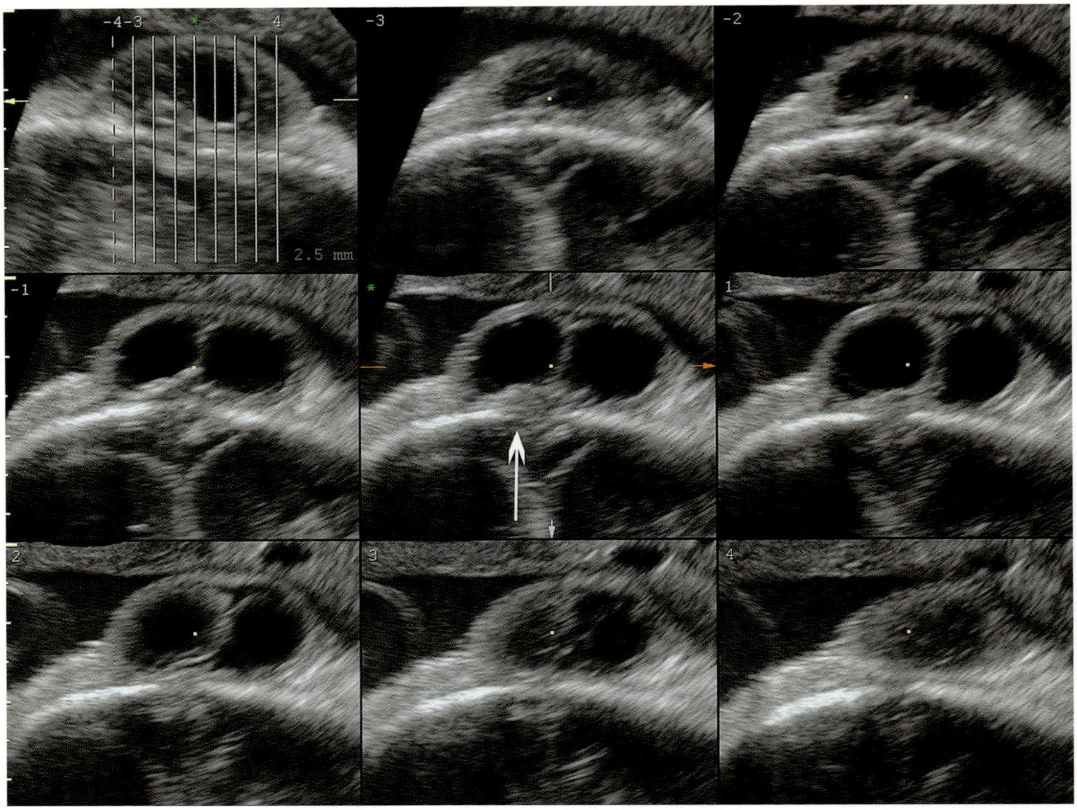

Fig. 24. Tomographic display demonstrating multiple successive views through a posterior cranial mass. Note the scull defect (*arrow*) through which the meninges protrude, confirming the diagnosis of a meningocele.

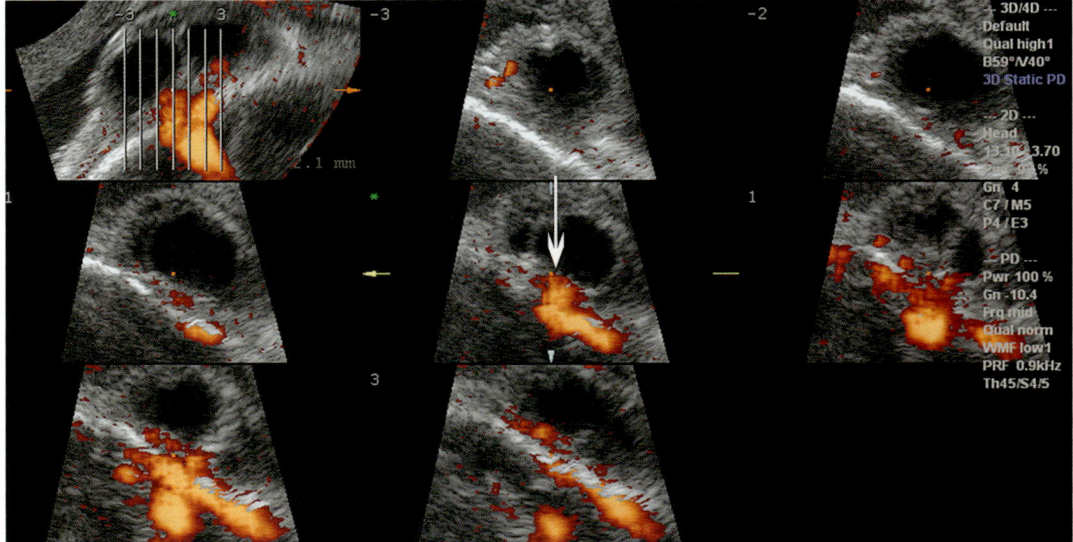

Fig. 25. Tomographic display mode with power Doppler angiography, demonstrating a blood vessel (*arrow*) traversing the scull defect and supplying the herniated meninges.

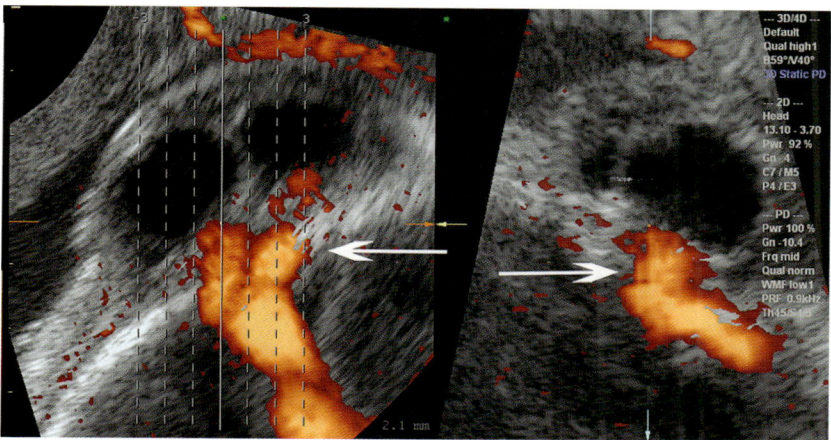

Fig. 26. A side-by-side Tomographic display view of the brain vessel (*arrows*) traversing the scull defect into the meningocele is shown in the coronal and axial views.

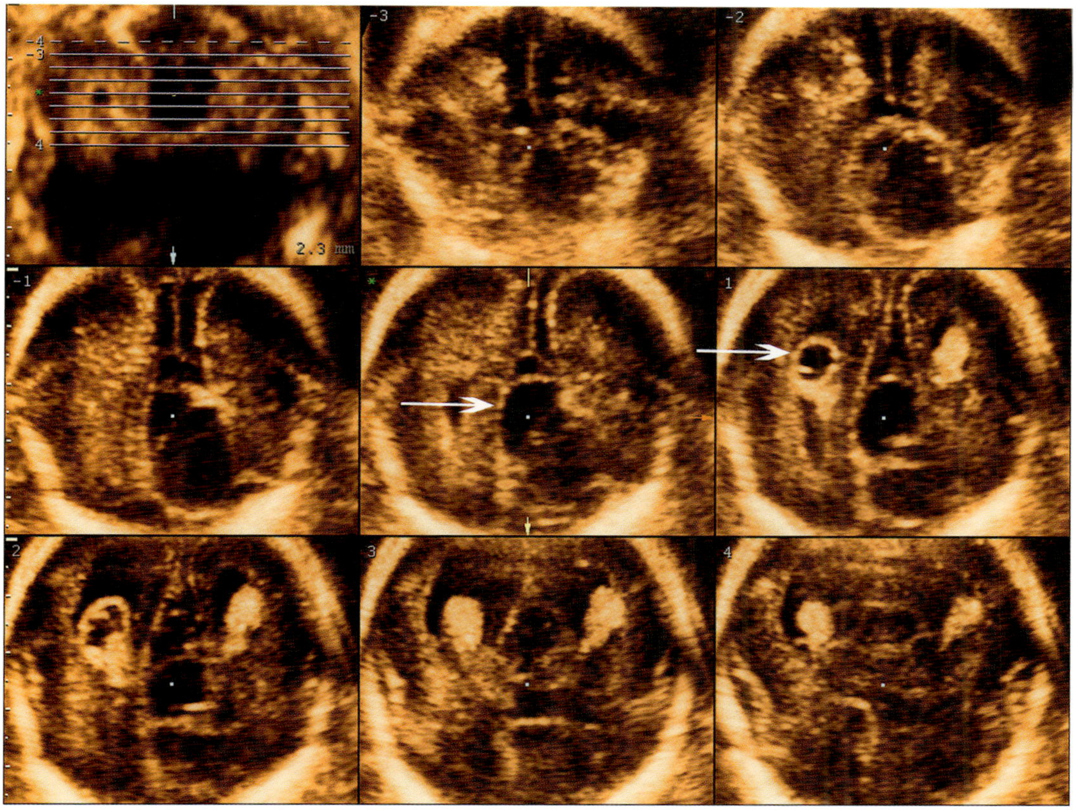

Fig. 27. Tomographic display mode, demonstrating multiple successive axial views through the entire height of the arachnoid cyst. The arrows point to the arachnoid cyst (Box *) and to a choroids plexus cyst (Box 1). Note the ventriculomegaly that is the result of pressure caused by the large arachnoid cyst.

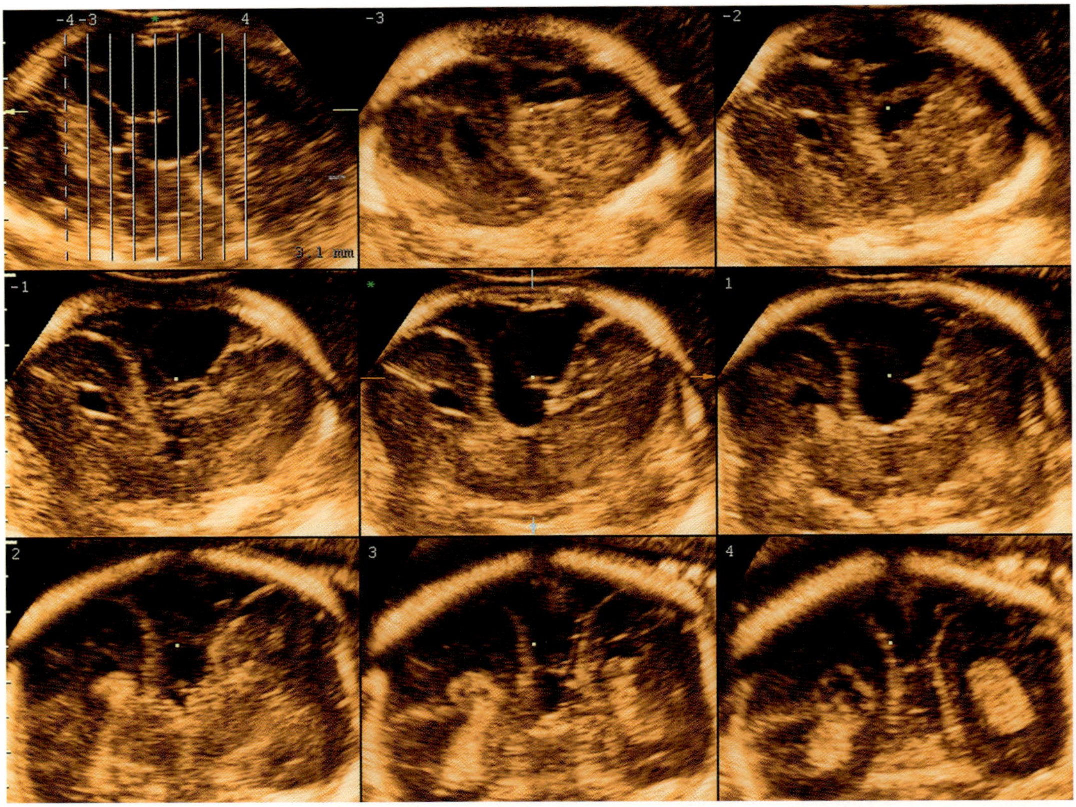

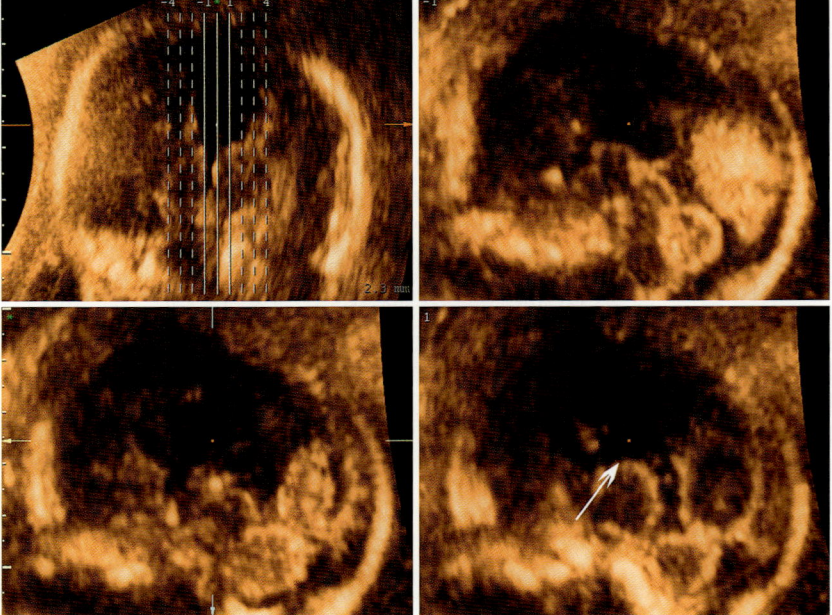

Fig. 28. Tomographic display mode, demonstrating multiple successive coronal views through the entire length of the arachnoid cyst, which is localized between the two brain hemispheres.

Fig. 29. Tomographic display mode, demonstrating multiple successive sagittal views through the entire width of the interhemispheric arachnoid cyst. The arrow points to the tela choroidea, which was considered to be the origin of this arachnoid cyst.

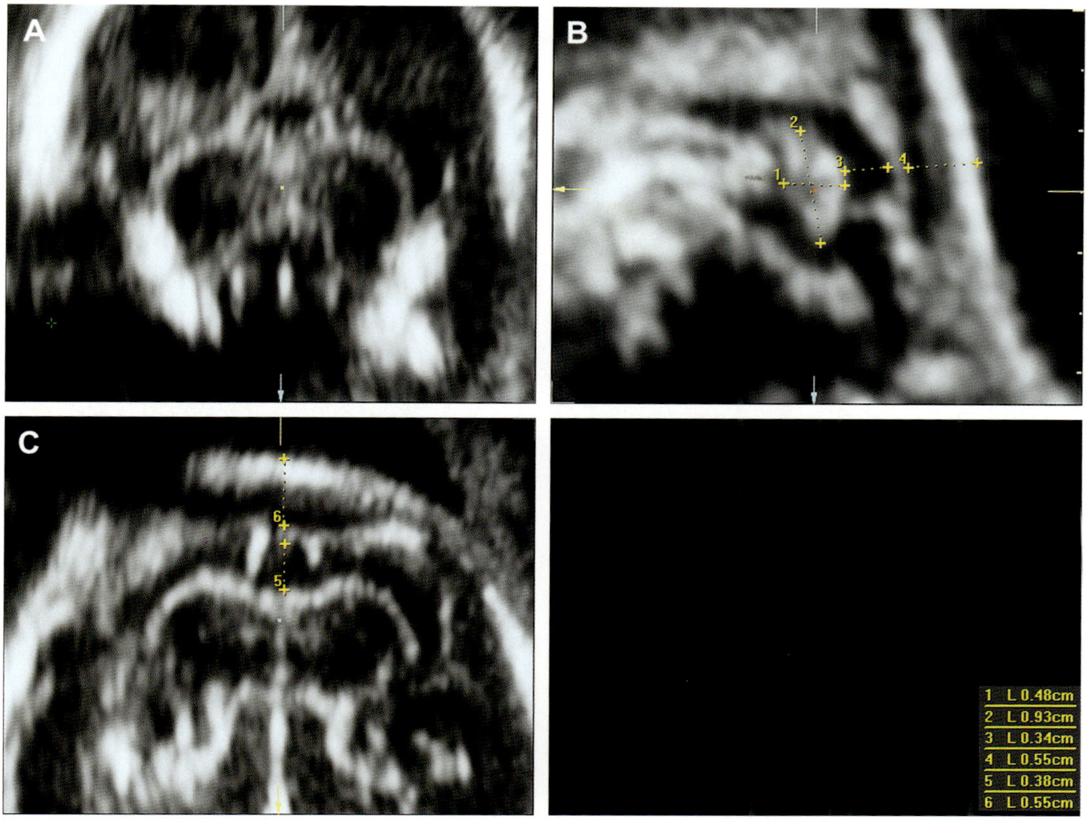

Fetal Neurosonology

Fig. 30. Multiplanar display of the posterior fossa. The cerebellum can be easily seen and measured on both the coronal plane (Box A) and the axial plane (Box C), demonstrating the entire cerebellar hemispheres. The median plane (Box B) provides additional information enabling the evaluation and measurement of the cerebellar vermis length (1) and height (2), the cisterna magna (3), and the nuchal fold (4). Measurements of the cisterna magna (5) and nuchal fold (6) are also seen on the axial plane in Box C. One should be aware of the fine linear echoes of the arachnoid, which are sometimes visualized in the cisterna magna. These lines (Box C) are normal and should not be confused with pathology.

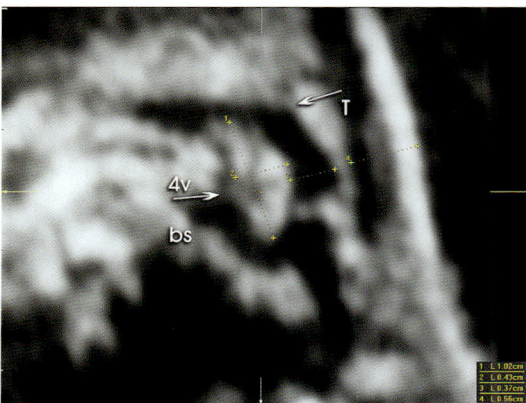

Fig. 31. Median plane focused on the posterior fossa, demonstrating measurements of the cerebellar vermis height (1) and length (2), cisterna magna (3), and nuchal fold (4). The different lobes of the cerebellar vermis can be identified in this plane. Additionally, the median plane can assist in the evaluation of the fourth ventricle (*arrow*, 4v), the relation of the vermis to the brain stem (bs), and the site and the position of the torcular (*arrow*, T).

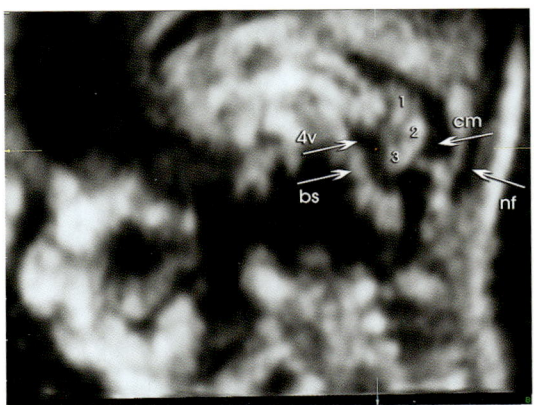

Fig. 32. Median plane of the fetal brain focused on the posterior fossa demonstrating the cerebellar vermis with its three lobes (marked as **1**, **2**, and **3**), the cisterna magna (cm), the nuchal fold (nf), the fourth ventricle (4v), and the brain stem (bs).

can indent the underlying cortex and mimic a picture of lissencephaly. As with other brain anomalies, the use of 3D ultrasound assists in the orientation of the lesion within the volume and can display it in a similar fashion to MR imaging, using the tomographic mode. **Figs. 27** to **29** demonstrate TUI display in different planes in a case of interhemispheric arachnoid cyst. The extent of the lesion, as well as its impact on the surrounding brain tissue, can be evaluated using the TUI mode in the different planes. The ability to display the images in tomographic slices facilitated the authors' understanding regarding the origin of the cyst, which appears to arise from the tela choroidea (**Fig. 29**, Box 1, *arrow*). Additionally, the 3D images and the possibility of slicing within the volume gave important clinical information to the pediatric neurosurgeon and played a practical role in counseling this patient.

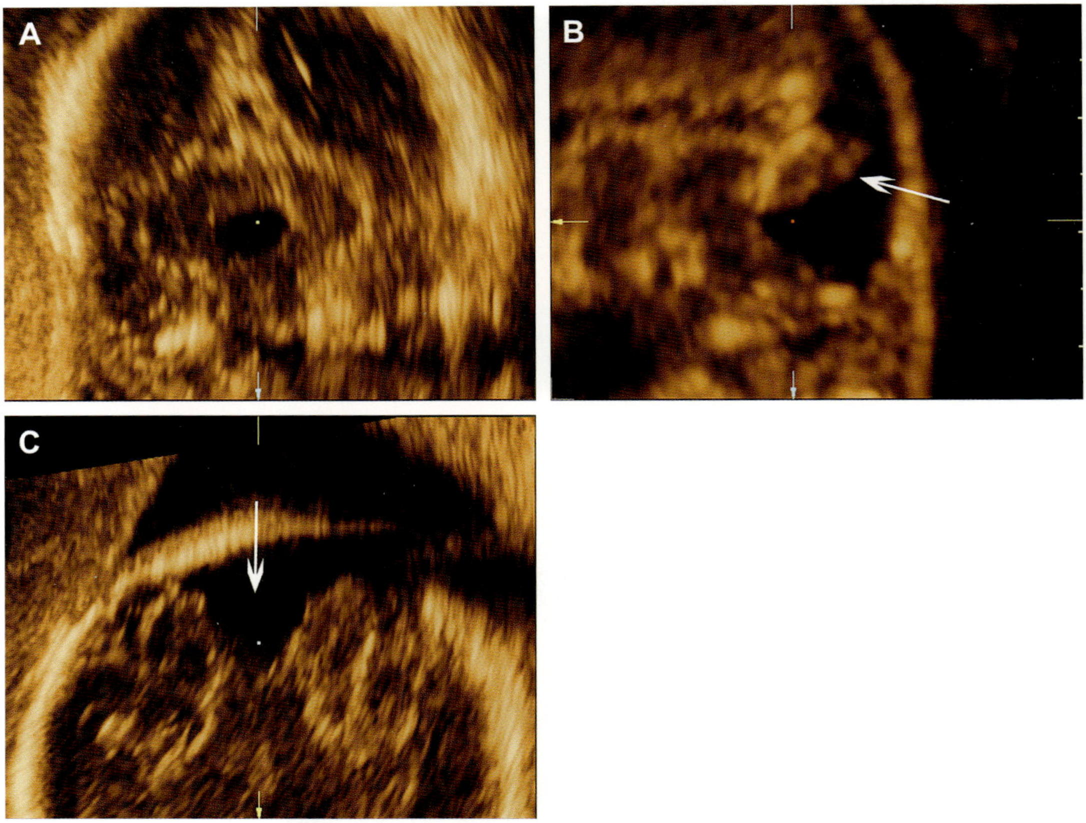

Fig. 33. Multiplanar display of a case of Dandy Walker malformation. The coronal plane (Box A) demonstrates the lateral displacement of the cerebellar hemispheres (splaying of the cerebellum). The median plane (Box B) is extremely informative, demonstrating the large posterior fossa cystic structure, the complete agenesis of the vermis, and the superior displacement of the tentorium and the torcular herophili (*arrow*). The axial view in Box C demonstrates the classic view of this anomaly, demonstrating the splaying of the cerebellum and the large cystic structure in the posterior fossa (*arrow*).

Posterior Fossa and Related Anomalies

Three-dimensional evaluation of the posterior fossa requires both technical expertise and understanding of the normal development of the fetal brain along gestation. Before 16 to 18 postmenstrual weeks, the cerebellar vermis is still not completely developed and the fourth ventricle clearly communicates with the cisterna magna through the widely open median aperture (foramen of magendie). Understanding the timing of vermian development is thus crucial to avoid misdiagnosis of posterior-fossa anomalies at this gestational age.

Traditionally, posterior-fossa anomalies have been diagnosed and classified based on the axial (transcerebellar) view (see **Fig. 14**c). However, many important features of the posterior fossa anatomy, such as the position of the vermis, tentorium, and the torcular (confluence of sinuses), cannot be adequately assessed using the axial view solely. Three-dimensional ultrasound enables the simultaneous evaluation of the three orthogonal planes of the posterior fossa (**Fig. 30**).

The median plane (**Figs. 31** and **32**) is especially important when establishing certain pathologies in the posterior fossa, as it depicts the size (height and length) and the orientation of the vermis, the cisterna magna, and the position of the torcular.

In the authors' experience, the best image of the posterior fossa can be obtained by aligning the tip of the transvaginal transducer with the posterior fontanelle. After acquisition of the volume in this manner, the posterior fossa can be evaluated using the coronal (occipital) plane, the traditional transcerebellar axial plane, and the median plane, which the authors' find extremely informative. Viñals and colleagues[21] reported the successful use of the volume contrast-imaging mode in the evaluation of the cerebellar vermis, which the authors' have also found useful.

The anomalies of the posterior fossa are a group of fluid-containing malformations that share few common features in their appearance and pathologic definition. This group includes several malformations (listed as most-to-least severe): Dandy-Walker malformation, Dandy-Walker

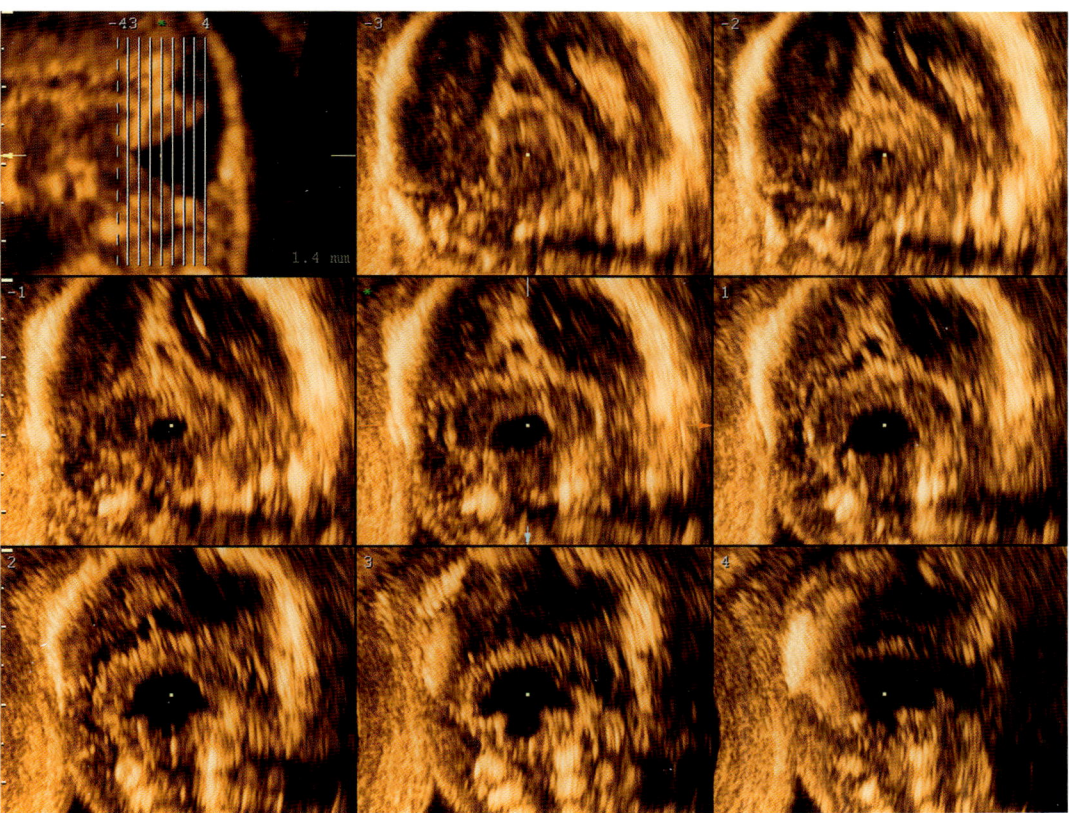

Fig. 34. Tomographic display mode demonstrating multiple successive coronal images taken throughout the length of the cerebellum. These views enhance our ability to evaluate the extent of the cerebellar anomaly.

variant, persistent Blake's pouch cyst, and mega cisterna magna. The previous confusing classification and nomenclature described the "Dandy-Walker continuum" and was based upon axial fetal ultrasound. It is now thought that a more accurate definition and description of these entities is required, because their pathogenesis, their anatomic picture, their prognosis, and their treatment are different. Therefore, the authors now approach these anomalies as different entities rather than a continuum, making the correct diagnosis extremely important. Differentiation between these malformations depends on the presence and the severity of the vermian hypoplasia, the presence or absence of posterior fossa cystic enlargement (the location of the torcular Herophili), abnormal communication between the fourth ventricle and the posterior fossa cyst, and the relationship between the position of the vermis and the brain stem. Three-dimensional ultrasound was found to be of significant assistance in the diagnosis of these different entities.[10] In the authors' experience this technique, especially if acquired with a high-frequency vaginal transducer through the posterior fontanelle, is extremely useful in achieving a "posterior-fossa window," enabling the evaluation of the posterior fossa and its relation with the brain stem. As described above, the multiplanar display mode can be used to easily detect the median plane. The authors consider it the plane of choice for evaluation of the vermis length and height, vermis position, and its relationship to the brain stem. When an anomaly is suspected, the median plane can further help in the evaluation of the size of the posterior fossa cyst, the superior displacement of the torcular Herephili, the configuration of the fourth ventricle, and measurement of the cisterna magna.

Dandy-Walker malformation

This severe malformation is characterized by an enlarged posterior-fossa fluid content and

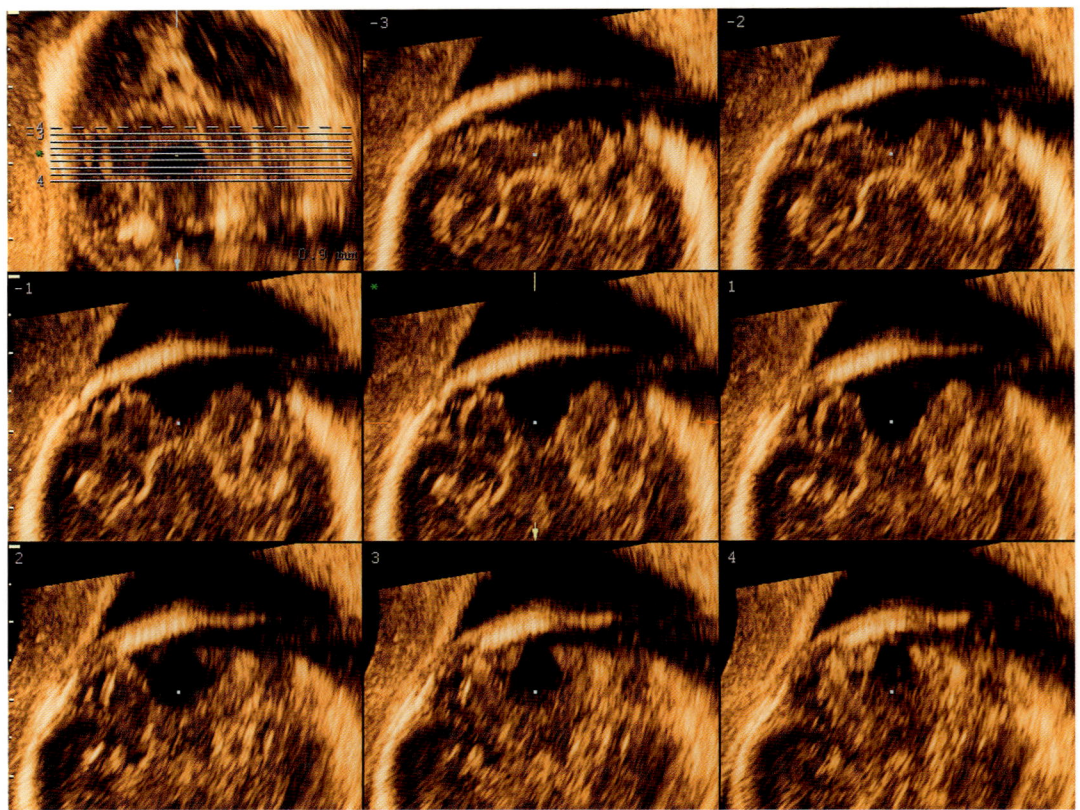

Fig. 35. Tomographic display mode, demonstrating multiple successive axial views taken through the entire height of the cerebellum. The lateral displacement of the cerebellar hemispheres can be evaluated at the different levels of the cerebellum.

a complete or partial agenesis of the vermis. The cerebellar hemispheres are laterally displaced (splaying of the cerebellum) and the tentorium and the torcular herephili are displaced superiorly (**Figs. 33–35**). In this case of Dandy Walker malformation, the multiplanar mode displays the extent of the anomaly, as it can be clearly identified on each one of the three orthogonal planes simultaneously. Despite the relative apparent sonographic findings, 20% to 40% of such cases are undetected antenatally. It is believed to have an incidence of 1 in 30,000 births, with most cases (50%–70%) associated with additional brain anomalies. In 50% to 70% of survivors, a poor neurodevelopment is observed. It is believed that isolated cases carry a recurrence risk of 1% to 5%.

Dandy-Walker variant
This anomaly consists of variable hypoplasia or agenesis of the vermis with or without enlargement of the cisterna magna, which communicates with the fourth ventricle. The cerebellar hemispheres maybe of normal size and frequently only subtle sonographic findings may be identified. At times, it is therefore a difficult prenatal sonographic diagnosis to make. An example of such a case can be seen in the multiplanar mode in **Fig. 36**.

Genetic factors play a major role in the etiology of both Dandy Walker malformation and variant. Agenesis of the vermis has been associated with a number of syndromes, such as Aicardi syndrome, chromosomal aneuploidy (trisomy 8 and 9, triploidy) as well as Fry, Meckel-Grubber, Neu-Laxova, Smith-Lemli-Opitz, and Walker-Warburg syndromes. Therefore, whenever these anomalies are detected, a genetic consultation and invasive genetic testing should be offered to the patient.

Persistent Blake's pouch cyst
This pathology is thought to result from failure of fenestration laterally through the lateral aperture (Luschka) and in the median plane through the

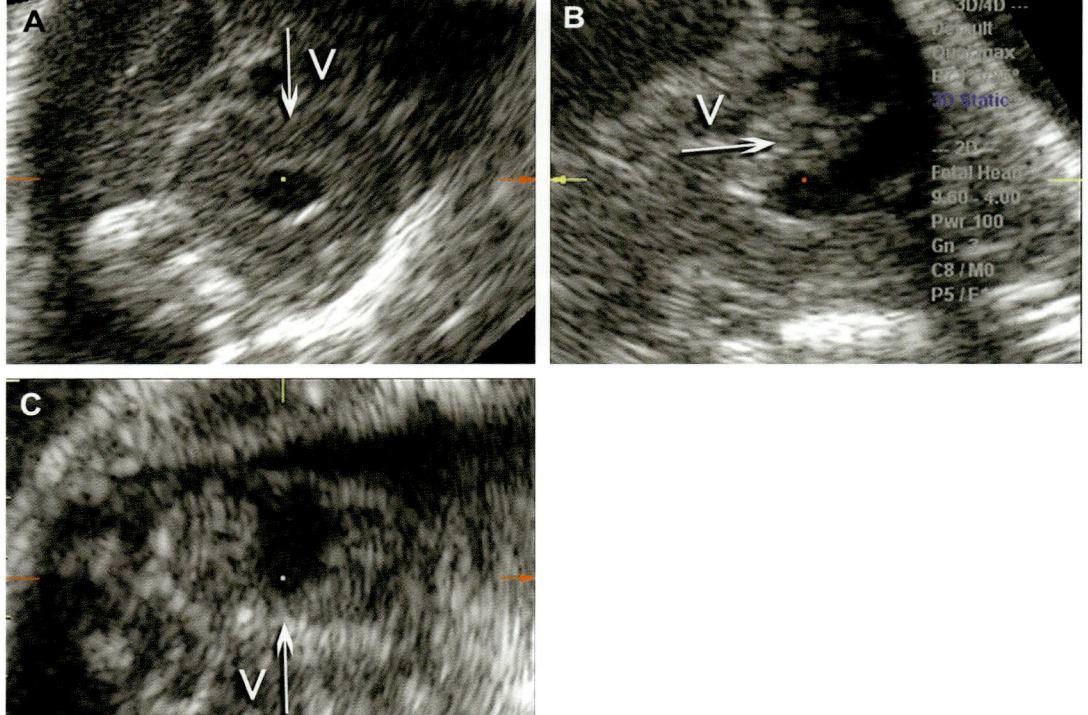

Fig. 36. Multiplanar mode of a fetus with Dandy Walker variant. Note the laterally displaced cerebellar hemispheres with the posterior fossa lesion seen in the coronal (Box A) and axial (Box C) views, respectively. Significant hypoplasia of the superiorly displaced vermis (*arrow*, V) can be seen as well as the enlargement of the cisterna magna, which is seen communicating with the fourth ventricle. The cerebellar hemispheres appear to be of normal size.

median aperture (Magendie), thereby preventing the connection and fluid drainage between the fourth ventricle "so called cyst" and the subarachnoid space (**Fig. 37**).

Sonographic diagnosis is possible because the cyst wall is evident on the axial and the sagittal planes. There is anechoic fluid inside the cyst and slightly low-level echoic fluid in the surrounding subarachnoid space. Additionally, the intact vermis may be displaced upward by the mass effect, which can also push the cerebellar hemispheres apart (splaying of the cerebellum), imitating some of the findings in cases of Dandy Walker malformation. Ventriculomegaly can sometimes be seen if the mass effect obliterates the cerebrospinal fluid drainage.

The prognosis is relatively good because postnatal shunting leads to re-expansion of the displaced brain structures.

Mega cisterna magna

This entity is characterized by an enlarged cisterna magna, measuring greater than or equal to 10 mm, with normally positioned and intact cerebellar vermis and fourth ventricle (**Fig. 38**). Its clinical significance as an isolated finding is uncertain, and no clear-cut prognostic data are available. These fetuses may be totally asymptomatic; however, some cases are associated with other malformations or chromosomal aberrations.

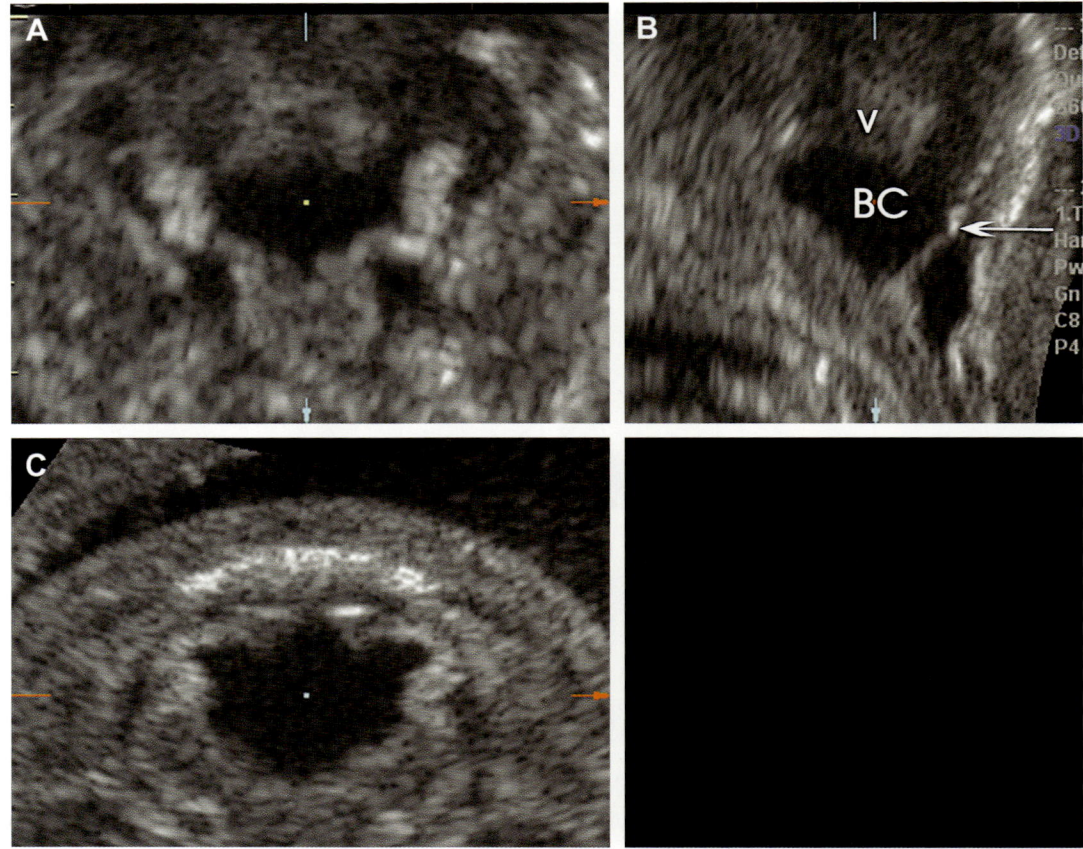

Fig. 37. Multiplanar mode of a case of Blake's pouch cyst. The cyst forms because of the accumulation of fluid in the fourth ventricle. The intact vermis can be seen on the sagittal plane in Box B (v), to be displaced upward by the mass effect. Additionally, the median plane assisted the authors in identifying the posterior cyst wall (*arrow*), as it is protruding into the cisterna magna. The Blake's pouch cyst is marked (BC) on the median plane in Box B. The coronal and axial views demonstrate splaying of the cerebellar hemispheres caused by the mass effect, as seen in Boxes A and C, respectively. In this case, without the image in the median plane, the diagnosis of Blake's pouch cyst would have been impossible.

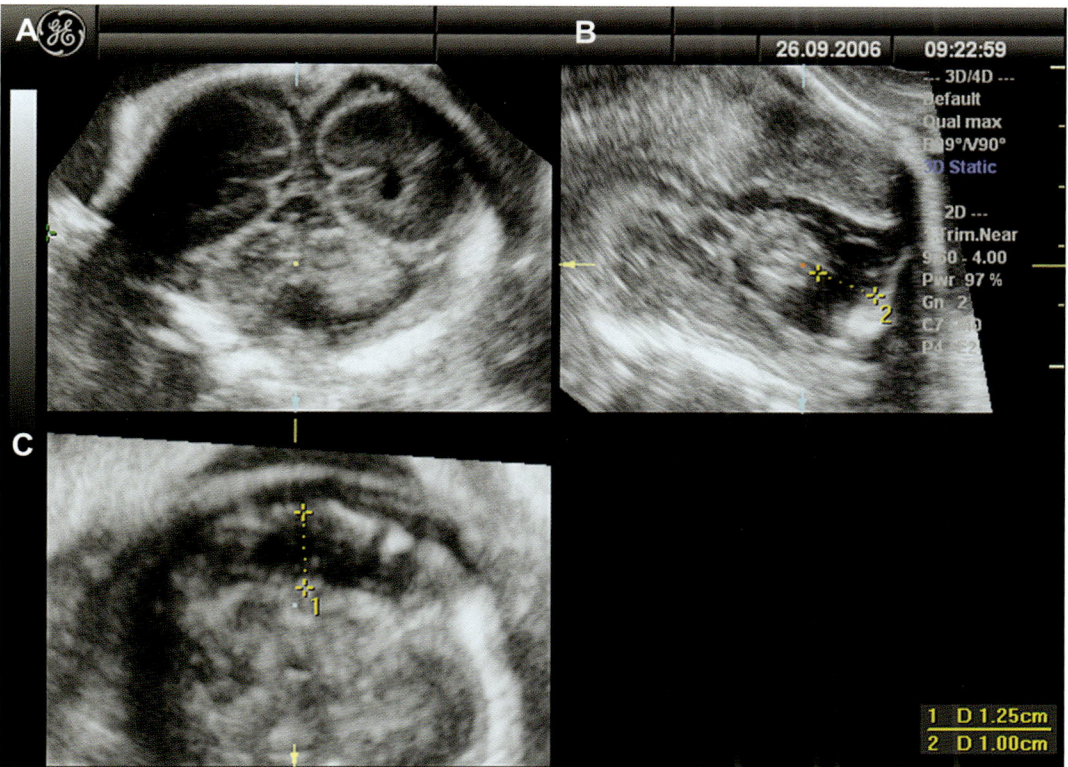

Fig. 38. Multiplanar mode of a brain in a fetus with mega cisterna magna. The characteristically enlarged cisterna magna can be seen on all three orthogonal planes (Boxes A, B, and C). Measurements are provided in this case in the median and the axial planes in Boxes B and C, respectively. Note the normally positioned and intact cerebellar vermis and fourth ventricle as seen on the median plane in Box B (*marked with the red marker dot*).

SUMMARY

In summary, the amazing technology of 3D imaging enables the examination of the fetal brain simultaneously in the three orthogonal planes, better defining the spatial relationship of brain structures and malformations. The authors routinely use the multiplanar mode to navigate through the brain volume, observing information on a specific structure in all three orthogonal planes. Other display options, mainly the tomographic mode, are used to display the anomaly. The varieties of display modes and the infinite number of different planes that can be generated facilitate the diagnostic process. Additional values of this technology include an off-line analysis of the volume by the sonographer or sonologist to obtain the necessary planes, as well as an electronic transmittal for an off-site expert to provide a second opinion consultation. This modality requires a short acquisition time, allowing high patient through-put and increased patient satisfaction. In addition, it is an excellent teaching tool and provides valuable information to consulting pediatric surgeons, plastic surgeons, neonatologists, neurologists and neurosurgeons.

REFERENCES

1. Goldstein I, Reece EA, Pilu G, et al. Sonographic evaluation of the normal developmental anatomy of the fetal cerebral ventricles. IV: The posterior horn. Am J Perinatol 1990;7:79–83.
2. Denkhaus H, Winsberg F. Ultrasonic measurement of the fetal ventricular system. Radiology 1979;131:781–7.
3. Cardoza JD, Goldstein RB, Filly RA. Exclusion of fetal ventriculomegaly with a single measurement: the width of the lateral ventricular atrium. Radiology 1988;169:711–4.
4. Goldstein I, Reece EA, Pilu G, et al. Sonographic evaluation of the normal developmental anatomy of the fetal cerebral ventricles. I: The frontal horn. Obstet Gynecol 1988;72:588–92.
5. Pilu G, Ghi T, Carletti A, et al. Three-dimensional ultrasound examination of the fetal central nervous system. Ultrasound Obstet Gynecol 2007;30(2):233–45.

6. International Society of Ultrasound in Obstetrics & Gynecology Education Committee. Sonographic examination of the fetal central nervous system: guidelines for performing the "basic examination" and the "fetal neurosonogram." Ultrasound Obstet Gynecol 2007;29(1):109–16.
7. Monteagudo A, Timor-Tritsch IE, Mayberry P. Three-dimensional transvaginal neurosonography of the fetal brain: "navigating" in the volume scan. Ultrasound Obstet Gynecol 2000;16(4):307–13.
8. Timor-Tritsch IE, Monteagudo A, Mayberry P. Three-dimensional ultrasound evaluation of the fetal brain: the three horn view. Ultrasound Obstet Gynecol 2000;16(4):302–6.
9. Correa FF, Lara C, Bellver J, et al. Examination of the fetal brain by transabdominal three-dimensional ultrasound: potential for routine neurosonographic studies. Ultrasound Obstet Gynecol 2006;27(5):503–8.
10. Pilu G, Segata M, Ghi T, et al. Diagnosis of midline anomalies of the fetal brain with the three-dimensional median view. Ultrasound Obstet Gynecol 2006;27(5):522–9.
11. Monteagudo A, Timor-Tritsch IE, Moomjy M. Nomograms of the fetal lateral ventricles using transvaginal sonography. J Ultrasound Med 1993;12:265–9.
12. Wang PH, Ying TH, Wang PC, et al. Obstetrical three-dimensional ultrasound in the visualization of the intracranial midline and corpus callosum of fetuses with cephalic position. Prenat Diagn 2000; 20(6):518–20.
13. Shapiro R, Galloway SJ, Shapiro MD. Minimal asymmetry of the brain: a normal variant. AJR Am J Roentgenol 1986;147:753–6.
14. Naidich TP, Schott LH, Baron RL. Computed tomography in evaluation of hydrocephalus. Radiol Clin North Am 1982;20:143–67.
15. Epstein F, Naidich T, Kricheff I, et al. Role of computerized axial tomography in diagnosis, treatment and follow-up of hydrocephalus. Child's Brain 1977;3: 91–100.
16. Noorani PA, Bodensteiner JB, Barnes PD. Colpocephaly: frequency and associated findings. J Child Neurol 1988;2:100–4.
17. Garg BP. Colpocephaly. An error of morphogenesis? Arch Neurol 1982;4:243–6.
18. Heinz ER, Ward A, Drayer BP, et al. Distinction between obstructive and atrophic dilatation of ventricles in children. J Comput Assist Tomogr 1980;3: 320–5.
19. Horbar JD, Heahy KA, Lucey JF. Ultrasound identification of lateral ventricular asymmetry in the human neonate. J Clin Ultrasound 1983;11:67–9.
20. Achiron R, Yagel S, Rotstein Z, et al. Cerebral lateral ventricular asymmetry: is this a normal ultrasonographic finding in the fetal brain? Obstet Gynecol 1997;89:233–7.
21. Viñals F, Muñoz M, Naveas R, et al. The fetal cerebellar vermis: anatomy and biometric assessment using volume contrast imaging in the C-plane (VCI-C). Ultrasound Obstet Gynecol 2005;26(6):622–7.

3D and 4D Fetal Neuroscan: Sharing the Know-how and Tricks of the Trade

Eran Bornstein, MD*, Ana Monteagudo, MD, Ilan E. Timor-Tritsch, MD

KEYWORDS

- 3D Ultrasound • 4D Ultrasound
- Fetal Brain • Neuroscan • Display modalities

We live in a 3D world. It is obvious, therefore, that visual information that is obtained from 2D images may be limited in reflecting the 3D structural reality. 2D ultrasonography (US) however, has been established as the mainstay of fetal brain sonographic evaluation. It was first obtained by means of conventional transabdominal scanning and, subsequently, the transvaginal-transfontanellar approach was developed, simulating the neonatal neuroscan and applying it to fetal brain imaging.[1–3] The addition of the transvaginal approach yielded high-resolution coronal and sagittal "slices" of any fetal organ but has been particularly helpful in fetal brain study.[4] The authors believe the separation of the two different approaches, the transabdominal and the transvaginal, has only historical significance. The two should be used jointly to obtain a complete fetal study if needed. The transvaginal study of the fetal brain, however, mandates additional experience, skills, and understanding of the structure or the brain malformation in question in order for diagnosticians to translate the 2D images to a reconstructed 3D model in their minds. Modern 3D techniques have emerged in recent years enabling acquisition of an entire volume of spatial ultrasound information that can be used in real time or stored for off-line analysis.[5] The volume can be analyzed and displayed in multiple planes and display modes that exceed by far the display capacities of 2D US and better reflect the 3D nature of the structure or anomaly in question.

The unique features of 3D US have helped bring the field of diagnostic fetal sonography to the next level. Until recently, similar 3D display modes were available only by the use of computed MR imaging . Thus, the use of 3D US in experienced hands may provide useful information that can be displayed without the need for high test costs, as MR imaging study is more expensive than fetal sonography. The authors believe that, in the near future, 3D evaluation of the fetal body, including the brain, will not be considered a separate entity or technique but rather an inherent part of fetal study in cases where congenital anomaly, specifically fetal brain abnormality, is suspected to obtain the utmost relevant information without which an examination would not be complete.

In the article by Bornstein and collegues, "The Utilization of 3D and 4D Dimensional Technology in Fetal Neurosonology", elsewhere in this issue, the use of 3D technology to study the normal and abnormal fetal brain is discussed; therefore, the fetal neuroscan imaging technique is referred to in this article. The value of this new and exciting technology is to supplement and enhance traditional 2D technology in appropriate cases rather than replacing it.

TECHNICAL ASPECTS

The physics aspect of 3D US technology and the different display modalities are beyond the scope

---

Division of Maternal Fetal Medicine, Department of Obstetrics & Gynecology, NYU School of Medicine, 550 First Avenue, Room 9N26, New York, NY 10016, USA
* Corresponding author.
E-mail address: eranbor@yahoo.com (E. Bornstein).

of this article. Several texts are available, however, for readers who are interested.[6,7]

With the improvement in gray-scale (2D) technology, excellent sectional images of the fetal body with its internal organs can be generated. Because 3D US data in the volume are obtained by a multitude of successive 2D US sectional images, these data can be used to reconstruct any desired plane by "slicing" the volume in various directions. Planes can be created that are virtually impossible to obtain by 2D scanning because of fetal position (abdominal probe) or limitations of the transducer (ie, when using a vaginal probe). With 2D scan alone, most of the time it is possible to obtain any two of the three classical planes (coronal, sagittal, and axial) of the fetal head or the brain; however, it is virtually impossible to obtain all three planes unless a fetus changes its position significantly during the scan.

Analysis of a 3D voxel-based volume (voxel is the smallest 3D US picture unit) allows a review of the volume in all directions and displaying it in the various display modes (**Fig. 1**).

The core part of the 3D system used, regardless of the differences in the display software, is the transducer. Most transabdominal and transvaginal transducers perform a mechanical sweep by an electrical motor that moves the crystal array in a certain range (angle of rotation). The planes are scanned in the volume at fixed and precise time intervals enabling an operator to make accurate measurements in the volume itself. The operator controls the quality of the image in the acquisition plane, the angle of rotation (section width), and the quality of the scan, which is dependent on the acquisition velocity. The final product of the processing module is displayed on the monitor and can be modified using the master control panel of the unit or stored as a volume, enabling future data manipulations.

Although 3D US is a static display of different planes within a volume of information, 4D US displays a continuously updated and newly acquired volume creating the impression of a moving structure. This is obtained by placing the region of interest (ROI) box over the structure to be scanned and initiating the scan. Initially, a real-time 2D US image appears on the monitor alongside a 4D US image. An operator then can manipulate the image using the X, Y, and Z axes to obtain the optimized rendered view and activate the full-screen display option to view the moving 3D image. The use of 4D US techniques while performing fetal neuroscan is not widespread and currently is limited to assessment of limb mobility.

DISPLAY MODALITIES

There are several ways of transforming voxel-based data to a 2D pixel-based image. Different manufacturers have software to analyze the 3D US volume, including 4D View (GE), QLAB (Phillips), SonoView Pro (Madison), and 3D Volume Viewer (Siemens). The various available software displays the scanning planes on the screen in different fashions. The descriptions, as well as the featured images in this article are the ones the authors prefer and have worked with over the years.

The Multiplanar or Orthogonal Display Mode

This specific display mode enables simultaneous display of an image in the three orthogonal planes. The acquisition plane appears in the upper left corner of the screen in box A. Box B displays the plane, which is perpendicular to the acquisition plane (A) but parallel to the ultrasound beam. Box C displays the reconstructed plane, which is perpendicular to the acquisition plane and the ultrasound beam. With some manipulation of the data volume, display of the three classical body planes (coronal, sagittal, and axial) can be achieved in these boxes. **Fig. 2** is an example of a multiplanar view of a normal brain displaying the three orthogonal planes (ie, coronal plane [box A], sagittal plane [box B], and axial plane [box C]). In the authors' experience and others', this modality provides the mainstay of 3D US evaluation of the fetal brain.[8–12] Not only can three orthogonal planes be seen simultaneously but also this display modality can be used to scroll through the volume,

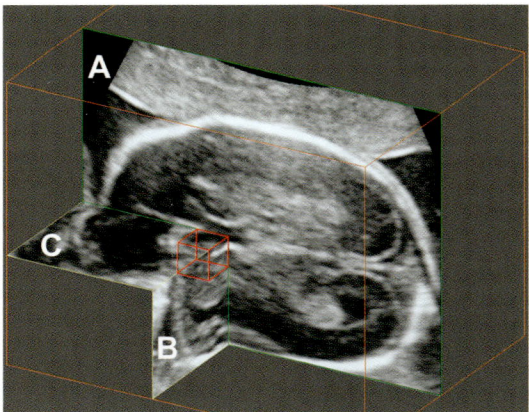

Fig. 1. 3D image of fetal head acquired in the axial plane (A) is presented in the niche mode. Plane B is perpendicular to plane A and parallel to the ultrasound beam and plane C is the reconstructed plane which is perpendicular to both planes (A and B). The red cubicle illustrates a voxel (the smallest unit of a 3D volume exactly as the pixel is the smallest unit of a 2D picture) placed at the point representing the transsection of the three orthogonal planes. The real size of a voxel is far smaller than the one displayed here.

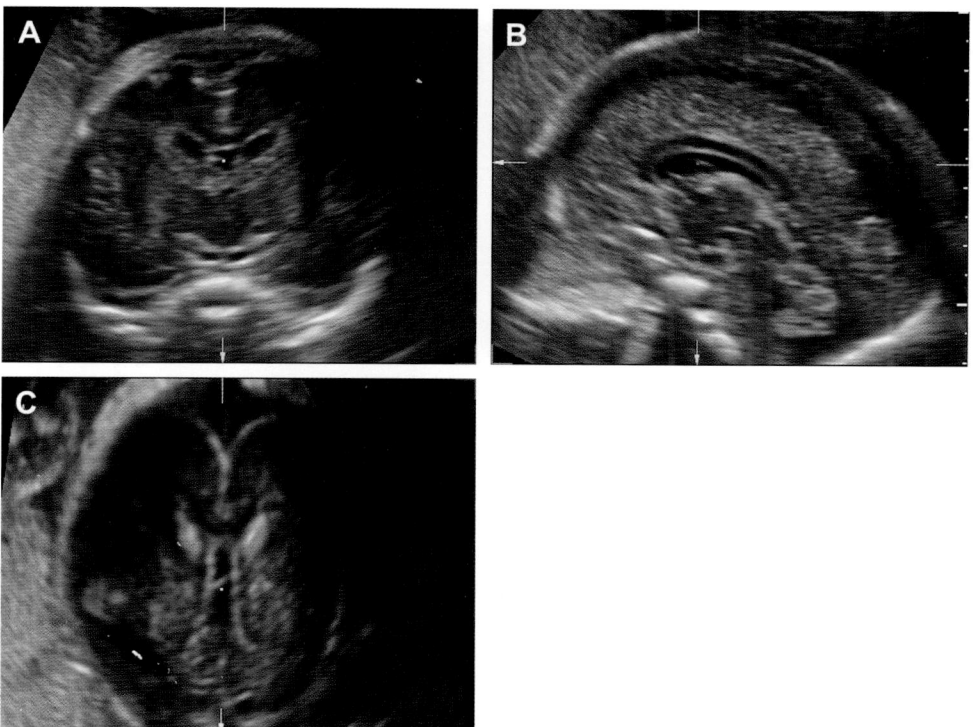

Fig. 2. Multiplanar display of the fetal brain in the three orthogonal planes: the coronal plane (*box A*), the median plane (*box B*), and the axial plane (*box C*). Note the marker dot representing the intersection of the three orthogonal planes, which is placed in this image in the cavum septi pellucidi.

as the planes can be moved back and forth, up and down, and from side-to-side within the volume. Thus, an operator can move freely (scroll or navigate) in the saved brain volume in all three planes to scrutinize it and obtain any desired diagnostic plane of the structure in question. An important tool used in this display modality is (what the authors call) the marker dot (see **Fig. 2**). This dot is generated by the intersection of the three orthogonal planes marking the same spot (or technically the same voxel) within the volume. The marker dot is freely movable by the operator, who can use it to pinpoint the same exact spot or structure on the three planes, which are being displayed simultaneously. For the authors, the liberal use of the marker dot constitutes the most valuable diagnostic feature of the software, enabling pinpointing the exact anatomic location of the structure of interest in one plane and having it displayed simultaneously in the other two orthogonal planes while navigating through the volume.

The Tomographic Ultrasound Imaging Mode

This mode displays an image in a successively sliced fashion, similar to the display in CT and MR imaging.[13] It probably is the most useful static display modality used during fetal neuroscan. Using the multiplanar mode to navigate through the volume and obtaining the desired plane, the tomographic mode then can be used to display consecutive sections of the area of interest in each one of the three orthogonal planes seen in boxes A, B, and C. The area of interest can be displayed as several reconstructed parallel 2D sections on a single panel. The operator has control over the thickness and the number of slices displayed. An additional option is to use the two-panel display in which the chosen plane is displayed side by side with the tomographic slice enabling navigation through both planes simultaneously. **Fig. 3** is an example of a tomographic view displaying successive (front-to-back) coronal sections of a normal fetal brain.

Inversion Mode

This unique modality, inversion mode, is a data manipulation that can be applied to the rendered volume to image sonolucent structures better. This technique inverts anechoic structures that are displayed as black on the customary 2D gray-scale ultrasound picture into a white, cast-like appearance (as in the negative of a film). This

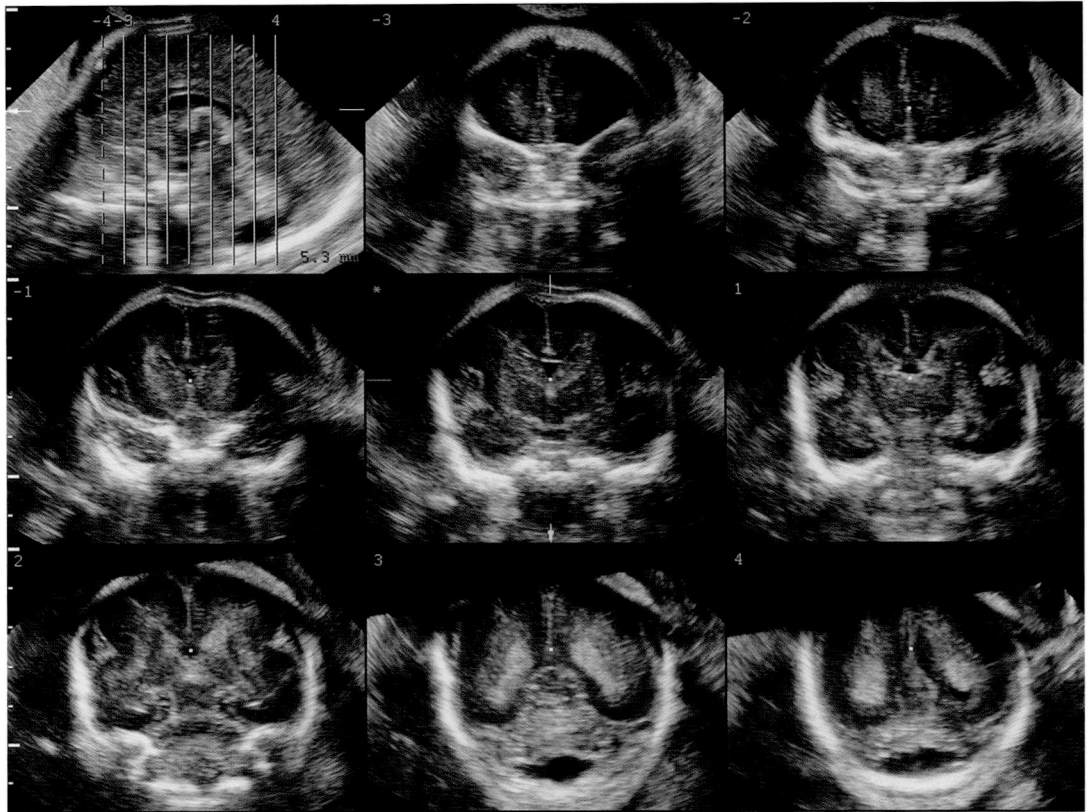

Fig. 3. Tomographic ultrasound image obtained on a fetal head in the sagittal position demonstrating successive coronal planes displayed from front to back. The coronal planes correspond to the planes that are marked crossing the brain on the sagittal image. The operator has control over the number and the thickness of the slices that are displayed as seen in the ultrasound image.

mode recently was described in the evaluation of the ventricular system in both—in normal cases studying the developing brain and in cases complicated by ventriculomegaly and holoprosencephaly.[14] The authors also have found this modality useful in such cases. **Fig. 4** demonstrates the use of the inversion mode to image the ventricular system in a fetus with hydrocephalus.

Thick-Slice Mode

The software collapses a preselected number of successive pictures (slices) and displays them in a 2D picture to enhance edge detection. The operator can adjust the slice thickness modifying the number of cuts that are compressed into the final rendered image. An example of a thick slice is presented in **Fig. 5**. This technique was further perfected and named volume contrast imaging (VCI) technology. The thick-slice technique still can be used; however, it requires several steps in contrast with the newer VCI, which is a one-step display mode.

Static Volume Contrast Imaging

VCI is a modality aimed at improving the resolution of the rendered image by displaying a thin slice of the acquired volume decreasing the ultrasound artifacts. By adding successive and defined number of tissue layers, ultrasound artifacts, such as speckles and noise pixels, are decreased or totally eliminated so that anatomic structures and their edges are enhanced, resulting in an increased contrast resolution. Several users apply the static VCI as a processing tool for the saved volume with a slice thickness of 1 to 3 mm as the modality of choice in analyzing the fetal brain.[12] **Fig. 6** enables comparison between traditional gray scale and VCI of the same brain image acquired in the axial plane.

Surface Rendering

Surface rendering is by far the most recognizable feature of 3D US and 4D US, which drew the initial attention of the industry, software developers,

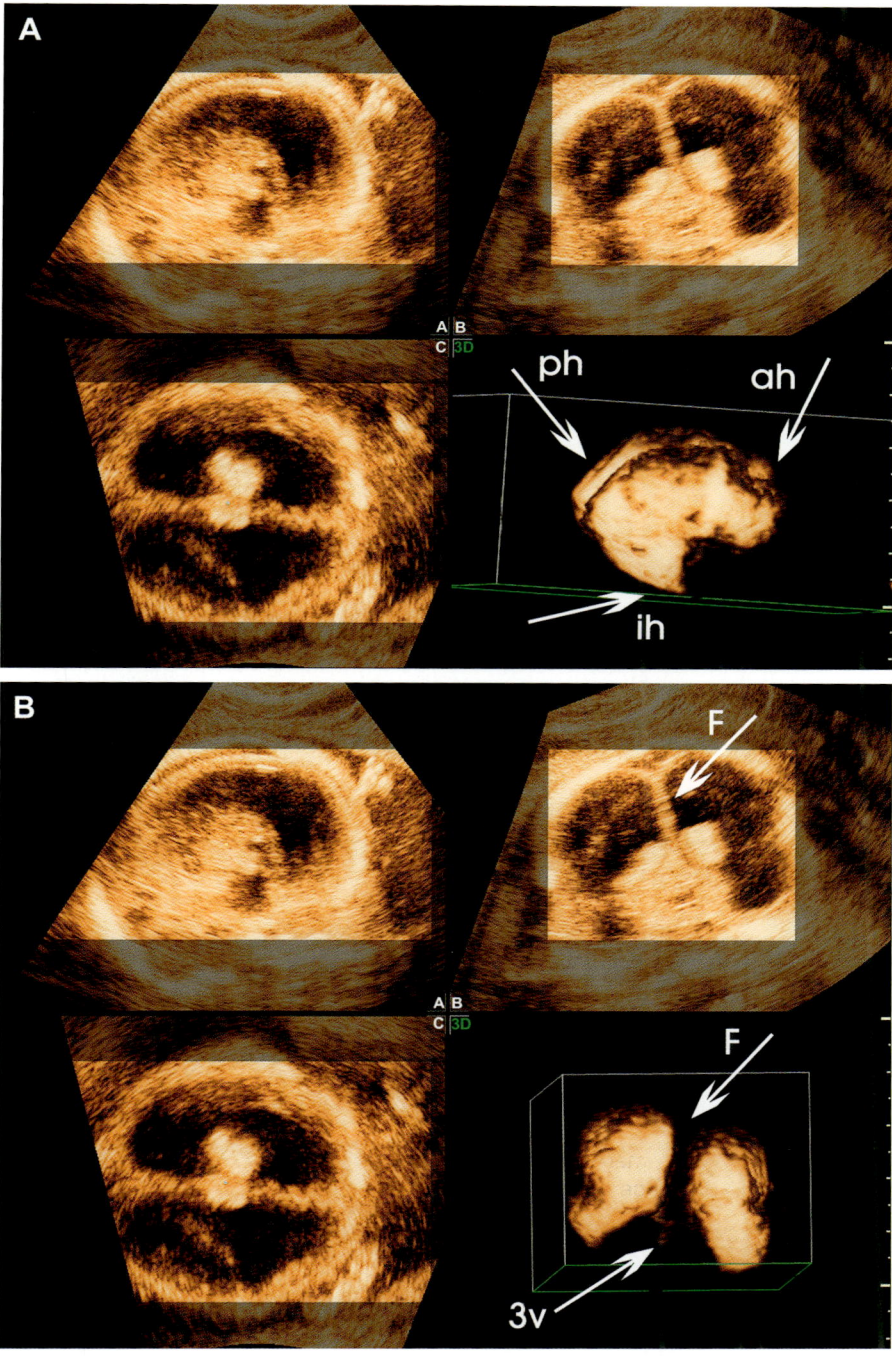

Fig. 4. These three images 4 A, B, and C are examples of the use of the inversion mode to image the fetal ventricular system in a case of hydrocephalus. This modality provides a cast-like pattern of the ventricular system. The inversion mode in Fig. 4A (*box 3D*) displays a sagittal view of the grossly dilated lateral ventricles. The arrows point to the anterior horn (ah), posterior horn (ph), and the inferior horn (ih). In Fig. 4B the inversion mode (*box 3D*) displays a posterior view of the dilated ventricular system. The falx (*arrow F*) can be seen as the black line separating the two lateral ventricles. The communication of the lateral ventricles with the third ventricle also can be seen (*arrow 3v*). The inversion mode in Fig. 4C (*box 3D*) demonstrates a view of the superior aspect of the lateral ventricles with a complete falx (*arrow F*) separating them. The falx (*arrow F*) and the dangling choroid plexus (*arrow cp*) also are seen on the coronal and axial planes in boxes B and C, respectively. The complete falx is important in this case to differentiate it from the various degrees of holoprosencephaly.

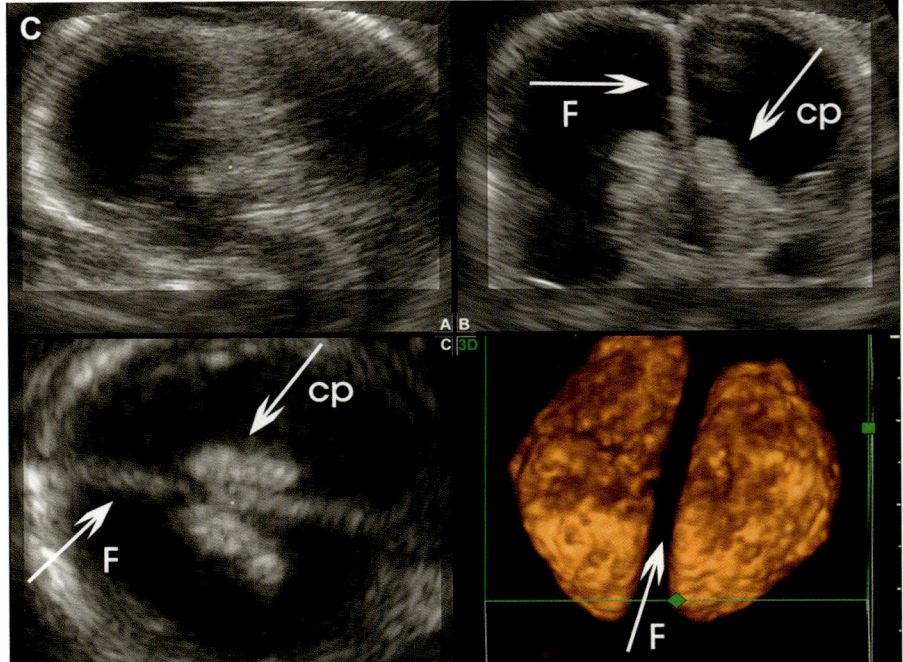

Fig. 4. (continued).

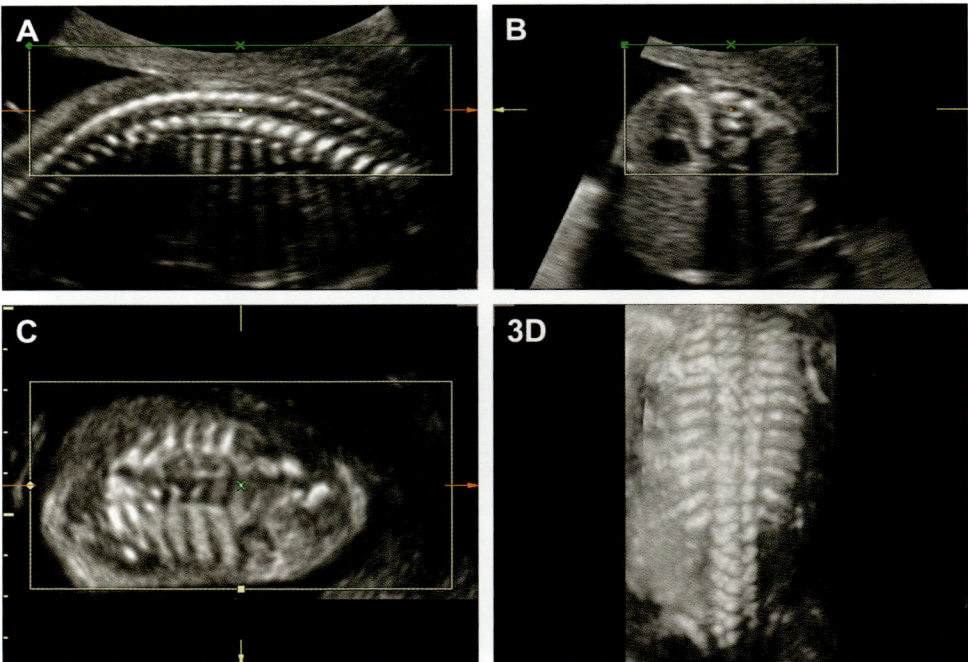

Fig. 5. Multiplanar mode of the fetal spine with the sagittal plane in (*box A*) and axial plane in (*box B*) demonstrating the complete vertebrae and the coronal longitudinal plane in (*box C*). The thick-slice technique was applied to obtain the rendered image in the maximum mode (*box 3D*). Using this technique, the slice thickness can be adjusted, controlling the numbers of slices that are compressed into the final rendered image.

3D and 4D Fetal Neuroscan

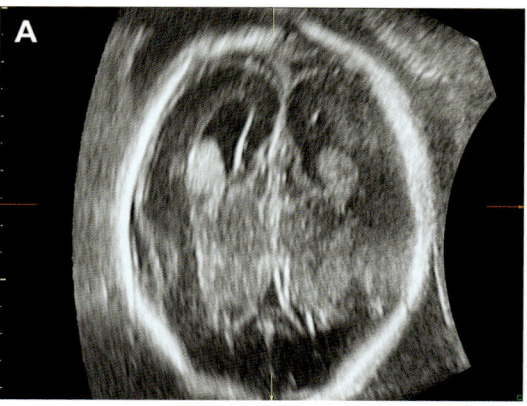
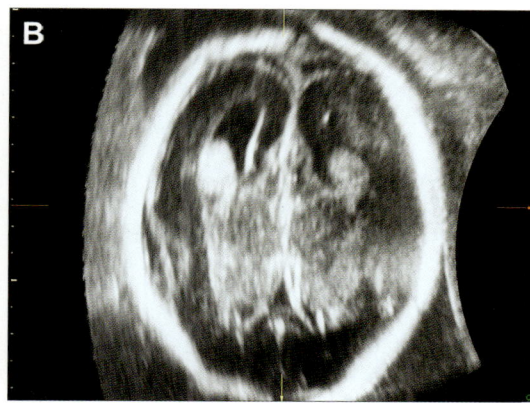

Fig. 6. Image enhancement software: comparison of the same image of a fetal brain in the axial transventricular plane is displayed in normal gray-scale (*A*) and in VCI mode (*B*). This modality may improve the resolution of the rendered image by displaying a thin slice of the acquired volume decreasing the ultrasound artifacts.

physicians, and patients to use of this technique. To obtain such an image, a well-defined interface (eg, tissue/fluid) is required. The volume then can be rotated in all three axes, X, Y, and Z, to achieve the right plane. The light mode of the surface rendering displays the body surface as it would appear if illuminated by a light source. This mode is not used frequently while imaging a brain during fetal neuroscan. It is an extremely useful mode, however, for detecting anomalies of the fetal face, which frequently are seen in cases of brain anomaly. **Fig. 7** demonstrates the use of surface rendering in the detection of unilateral cleft lip.

Transparency Mode

This modality, transparency mode, also called the x-ray mode or the maximum mode, was designed to retain only strong US echoes. Because weaker tissue echoes are suppressed and the bones usually provide the strongest echoes, images resemble x-ray pictures. This mode is helpful particularly for enhancing the evaluation of the skull in cases of microcephaly; skull defect, such as cephalocele; abnormality of the skull sutures; and evaluation of the fetal skeleton (eg, in examining the spine for neural tube defects). **Fig. 8** demonstrates the entire fetal spine and rib cage rendered in the maximum mode. Imaging the ribs can assist in localizing the precise level of vertebrae associated with the spine anomaly, thus having an important prognostic role.

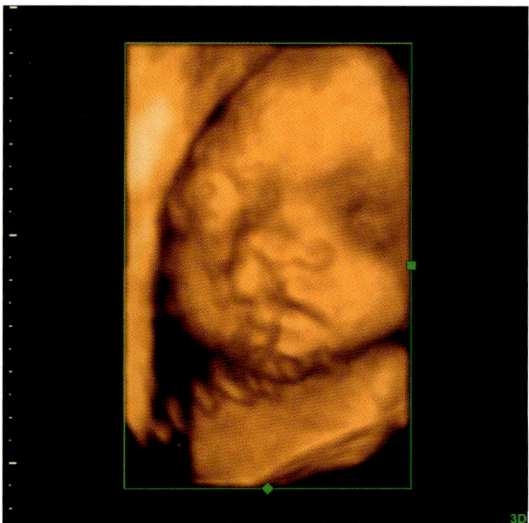

Fig. 7. Surface rendering of the fetal face demonstrating unilateral cleft lip.

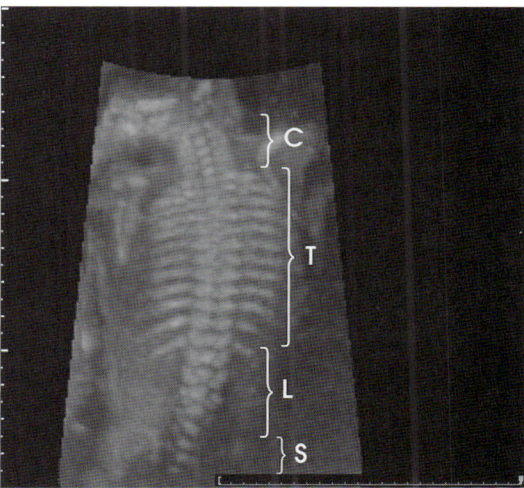

Fig. 8. The entire fetal spine and rib cage is displayed in this image, which was rendered in the transparency (maximum) mode. The evaluation of the fetal bony structures can be enhanced with this mode by providing precise localization of the exact level of the vertebra. The marked area shows the cervical spine (C), thoracic spine (T), lumbar spine (L), and sacrum (S).

3D Angiography

Similarly to using 2D gray-scale ultrasound, power angiography or color Doppler mode detects blood flow and can be used while acquiring a 3D US volume. These are useful imaging options of 3D US equipment while performing fetal brain scanning.[15–17] In selected cases, volume scans can be obtained using power angiography to image various main vessels in the brain. The authors are interested mainly in the course of the pericallosal branch of the anterior cerebral artery. The course of this vessel and its branches are demonstrated in **Fig. 9**. The technique of volume acquisition and manipulation is the same as with other 3D US modes. This mode of the 3D US machine may assist tracing a deviant course of any artery through the combined use of power angiography and the marker dot. Another common helpful use of power Doppler while performing fetal neuroscan is imaging the circle of Willis. The clinical importance of this technique is largely in cases where a middle cerebral artery Doppler study is required. **Fig. 10** displays a multiplanar mode using the thick-slice technique to image the circle of Willis.

SPECIAL CONSIDERATIONS OF 3D FETAL ULTRASOUND

The advantages and disadvantages of 3D ultrasound in general and during fetal neuroscan in particular have to be considered.

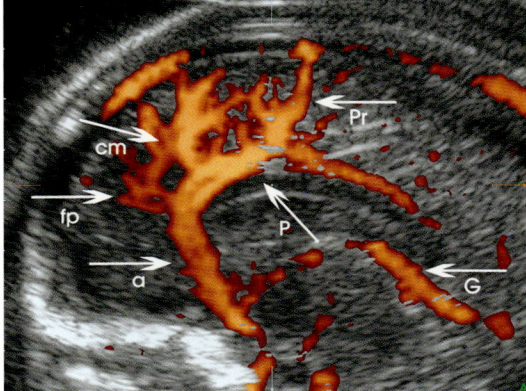

Fig. 9. 3D volume acquired with power Doppler positioned at the median plane demonstrating the branching of the complete pericallosal artery from the anterior cerebral artery. The presence of the entire pericallosal artery confirms the presence of a normal corpus callosum. The arrows point to the anterior cerebral artery (a), frontopolar artery (fp), callosomarginal artery (cm), the pericallosal artery (P), the precuneal artery (pr), and the vein of Galen (G).

Advantages of 3D Ultrasound

1. As described previously, the major advantage of 3D US is the ability to view a structure or organ of interest simultaneously in the three perpendicular planes, rotate the image, and freely navigate through the volume in endless options of angles. This enhances the assessment of malformations by allowing images to be resliced and viewed from angles that are not available with 2D imaging alone and display them tomographically in fashion similar to CT and MR imaging.
2. The volume can be stored for future off-line evaluation, enabling further manipulations, reslicing, and displaying modes not performed at the time of examination or initial evaluation.
3. Electronic means of communication enable sending the volumes to specialists anywhere in the world for second-opinion evaluation or consultation. Recipients then can manipulate the volume independently to obtain the desired sections and planes. The authors have been using this advantage successfully in the past few years by providing consultations to several colleagues after reviewing the volumes they saved in an Internet-based file transfer protocol.
4. Another advantage is that the surface-rendering mode produces an image similar to a photograph, which is especially useful in patient education and counseling. Patients viewing a small fetal omphalocele, encephalocele, or facial abnormality, such as a cleft lip, may be better informed as they note the appearance and size of the anomaly. The same applies for medical consultants, such as pediatric surgeons, neurosurgeons, and plastic surgeons, who may obtain important clinical information regarding the in utero anomaly, assisting them in early counseling of patients and planning postpartum management before a fetus is born. **Fig. 11** is a multiplanar mode with surface rendering of a unilateral cleft lip. This image provides reassurance to parents and plastic surgeons as to the extent of an anomaly and the likely favorable cosmetic prognosis.
5. Scanning time may be reduced significantly with 3D US scanning allowing processing the volume after a patient has left the examination suite. This may result in a better safety profile because of reduced exposure time, allowing for more efficient use of staff and equipment and increased patient satisfaction.
6. Positive influence on maternal-fetal bonding has been described after obtaining 3D US.[18]

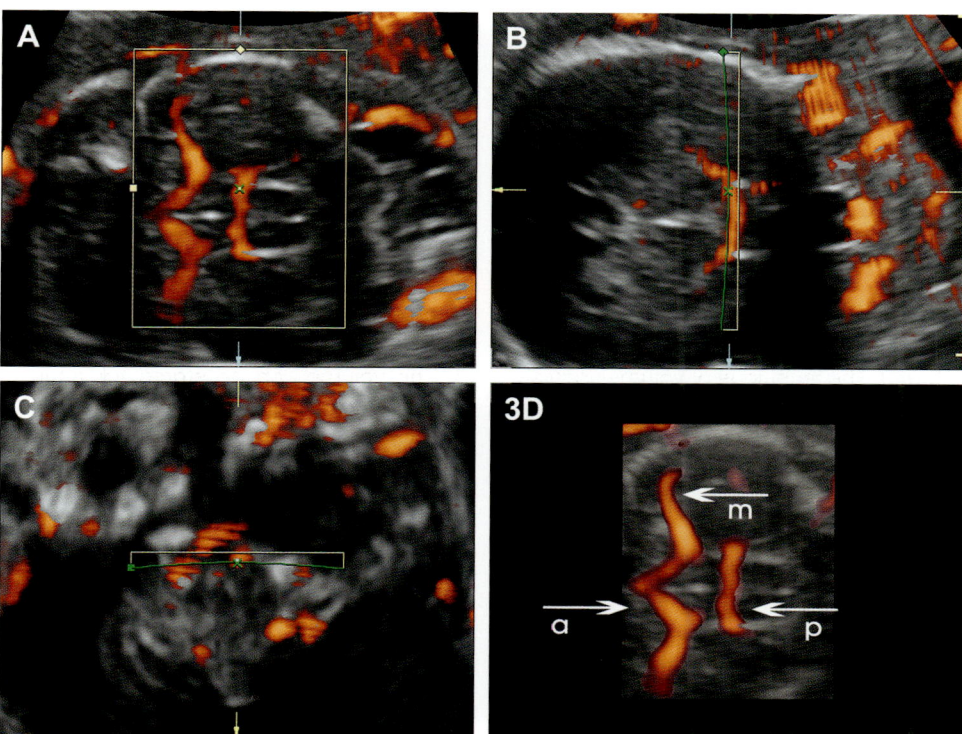

Fig. 10. The use of power Doppler is shown in this multiplanar image demonstrating the circle of Willis on the axial plane (*box A*). Thick-slice technique was used to obtain a rendered image of the circle of Willis (*box 3D*). The arrows point to the anterior cerebral artery (a), middle cerebral artery (m), and the posterior cerebral artery (p).

Specific Advantages of 3D Ultrasound During Fetal Neuroscan

1. The main advantage of 3D US in performing a fetal neuroscan, in the authors' experience, is the use of the multiplanar orthogonal display mode to navigate through the volume. By doing so, views can be obtained that are impossible (or extremely difficult) to obtain by traditional 2D US. As discussed previously, after achieving the specific plane using this technique, additional display modes can be applied to obtain a diagnostic image with the tomographic mode the most useful during the fetal neurosonogram.
2. The sections recreated from the 3D US volume are parallel to each other and do not radiate from a common point (the fontanelle) as is the case in conventional 2D transvaginal transfontanellar neurosonography and neonatal neuroscan. This makes 3D scanning of the fetal brain similar to conventional imaging using CT and MR imaging. **Fig. 12** demonstrates the different angles in which the coronal views are obtained with transvaginal neuroscan and with 3D reconstruction, respectively.
3. As discussed previously, the power angiography mode can be used in selected cases to obtain a volume imaging of various main vessels in the brain. The authors are interested mainly in the course of the pericallosal branch of the anterior cerebral artery. In cases of space-occupying lesions, the anatomy of the vessels may be of use in determining the size and extent of the lesion. In cases of brain tumor, its vascularity helps to evaluate the nature of the lesion. Using 2D US to obtain the "perfect" median (midsagittal) plane requires experience in transvaginal brain scan and at times may not be obtained because of unfavorable fetal position or presentation. Manipulating the 3D US to obtain the "perfect" median plane can be achieved easily by aligning the axial and coronal planes in the right position (discussed later). In some cases, in which the artery deviates from the midline because of pressure from a structure (such as a cyst), the course of the displaced artery can be followed using 2D US scans only with great difficulty or not at all. 3D angiography may assist in tracing the deviant course of the artery with the combined use of the marker dot.

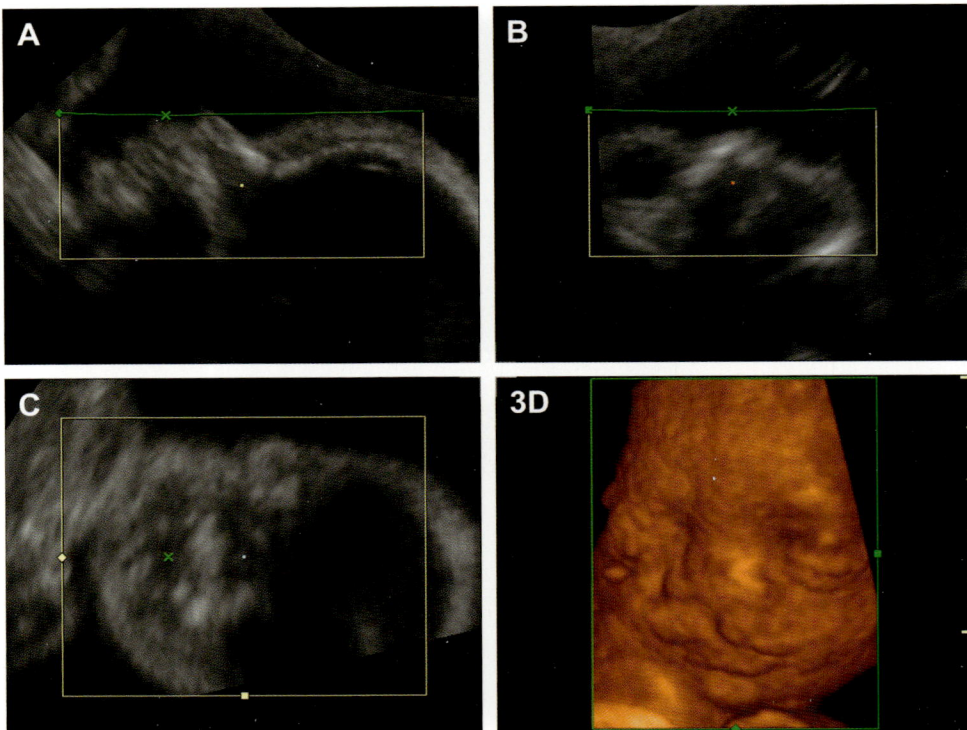

Fig. 11. Multiplanar image of fetal face after manipulation of the volume to display the fetal profile in box A. A unilateral cleft lip is seen in the 3D rendered box. This image may assist the plastic surgeon in counseling the patient and planning the postpartum management before the baby is born.

Limitations of 3D Ultrasound

1. In general, the limitations of 3D US are few and mainly reflect lack of adequate experience because of its long learning curve.[19]
2. The quality of an image displayed in the orthogonal planes (or any other render or display) can be only as good as the 2D US image in the acquisition plane. In addition, the reconstructed third plane (C plane) always will have lower resolution and an increased level of artifacts. The quality may be improved somewhat by using the thick-slice or the VCI application (discussed previously).
3. Acoustic shadowing in 2D US image in the acquired plane results in fixed acoustic shadow also limiting the 3D volume. For example, a 2D US image of the fetal brain obtained through the occipital bone may have poor quality of the intracranial structures as the thick bone creates an acoustic shadow. Similarly, a 3D volume obtained in this manner includes this fixed acoustic shadow embedded in the volume. Therefore, the prerequisite for a good 3D US image is to generate good-quality 2D US image.
4. Fetal motion is a major limitation causing artifacts that may preclude the acquisition of a good 3D US volume making it necessary to obtain additional volumes. This usually is overcome by decreasing the acquisition time of the volume using the low- or medium-quality sweep and by obtaining the volume in a time period with no fetal or maternal movements. The authors frequently instruct patients to hold their breath at the time of volume acquisition to limit any possible movement. This is true for volumes requiring long acquisition times, such as those containing color or power Doppler information.
5. The surface-rendering mode requires a fluid-tissue interface that sometimes may be compromised by an unfavorable fetal position, a fetal hand over the fetal face, or a fetal face too close to the anterior placenta. The electronic scalpel or the lectronic eraser may assist in eliminating structures that are not desired or that block the target structure.
6. Additional drawbacks that apply to 3D US just as in 2D US are the difficulty of obtaining a good image in patients who are obese or present with oligohydramnios and a nonfavorable

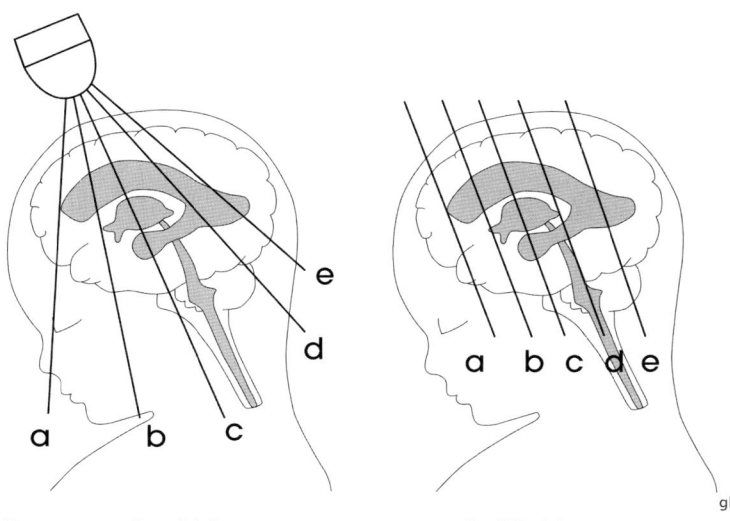

Fig. 12. The diagrams demonstrate the different angles in which the coronal views are obtained with transvaginal and with 3D neuroscans, respectively. The sections recreated from the 3D volume are parallel to each other and not radiating from a common point (the anterior fontanelle) as is the case with conventional 2D transvaginal neurosonography and neonatal neuroscan.

fetal position limiting the acquisition of the volume.

7. 3D US requires more expensive, updated ultrasound machines and software and is regarded as experimental by most health care carriers. For now, its use is limited by availability, financial aspects, and inexperienced users.

Limitations Unique to the 3D Neurosonogram

Specific limitations to the use of 3D US during fetal neuroscan are few. Generally, a high-frequency transvaginal ultrasound probe produces better images with higher resolution. The fetus must be in vertex presentation and the probe should be directed to perform a transvaginal transfontanellar neuroscan. In cases of breech presentation, acquisition of the volume should be attempted through the fontanelles, the sutures, or the thinner temporal bone to obtain a better view of the intracranial structures. At times, external version of the fetus into vertex presentation is warranted in fetuses with strong suspicion of a brain anomaly. Imaging the posterior fossa may be compromised by the acoustic shadow of the thick petrous ridge of the skull limiting the ability to image the brainstem. Volume acquisition through the posterior fontanelle or the posterior section of the sagittal suture may assist in overcoming this problem. Another limiting factor is the rare case of craniosynostosis in which the early fusion of the sutures limits easy scanning access to the brain that may be partially overcome by using the higher-frequency transvaginal transducer.

REFERENCES

1. Monteagudo A, Timor-Tritsch IE, Moomjy M. Nomograms of the fetal lateral ventricles using transvaginal sonography. J Ultrasound Med 1993;12:265–9.
2. Monteagudo A, Timor-Tritsch IE, Moomjy M. In utero detection of ventriculomegaly during the second and third trimesters by transvaginal sonography. Ultrasound Obstet Gynecol 1994;4:193–8.
3. Timor-Tritsch IE, Monteagudo A. Transvaginal fetal neurosonography: standardization of the planes and sections used by anatomic landmarks. Ultrasound Obstet Gynecol 1996;8:42–7.
4. Goldstein I, Reece EA, Pilu G, et al. Sonographic evaluation of the normal developmental anatomy of the fetal cerebral ventricles. IV: the posterior horn. Am J Perinatol 1990;7:79–83.
5. Gonçalves LF, Lee W, Espinoza J, et al. Three- and 4-dimensional ultrasound in obstetric practice: does it help? J Ultrasound Med 2005;24(12):1599–624.
6. Baba K, Jurkovic D. Three-dimensional ultrasound in obstetrics and gynecology. The Parthenon Publishing Group; 1997.
7. Nelson TR, Downey DB, Pretorius DH, et al. Three-dimensional ultrasound. Philadelphia: Lippincott, Williams & Wilkins; 1999.
8. Mueller GM, Weiner CP, Yankowitz J. Three-dimensional ultrasound in the evaluation of fetal head and spinal anomalies. Obstet Gynecol 1996;88:372–8.
9. Timor-Tritsch IE, Monteagudo A, Mayberry P. Three-dimensional ultrasound evaluation of the fetal brain: the three horn view. Ultrasound Obstet Gynecol 2000;16(4):302–6.

10. Correa FF, Lara C, Bellver J, et al. Examination of the fetal brain by transabdominal three-dimensional ultrasound: potential for routine neurosonographic studies. Ultrasound Obstet Gynecol 2006;27(5):503–8.
11. Pilu G, Segata M, Ghi T, et al. Diagnosis of midline anomalies of the fetal brain with the three-dimensional median view. Ultrasound Obstet Gynecol 2006;27(5):522–9.
12. Pilu G, Ghi T, Carletti A, et al. Three-dimensional ultrasound examination of the fetal central nervous system. Ultrasound Obstet Gynecol 2007;30(2):233–45.
13. Monteagudo A, Timor-Tritsch IE, Mayberry P. Three-dimensional transvaginal neurosonography of the fetal brain: 'navigating' in the volume scan. Ultrasound Obstet Gynecol 2000;16(4):307–13.
14. Kim MS, Jeanty P, Turner C. Benoit B. Three-dimensional sonographic evaluations of embryonic brain development. J Ultrasound Med 2008;27(1):119–24.
15. Pooh RK, Pooh K. Transvaginal 3D and doppler ultrasonography of the fetal brain. Semin Perinatol 2001;25(1):38–43.
16. Pooh RK, Pooh KH. The assessment of fetal brain morphology and circulation by transvaginal 3D sonography and power doppler. J Perinat Med 2002;30(1):48–56.
17. Chang CH, Yu CH, Ko HC, et al. Three-dimensional power doppler ultrasound for the assessment of the fetal brain blood flow in normal gestation.
18. Ji EK, Pretorius DH, Newton R, et al. Effects of ultrasound on maternal-fetal bonding: a comparison of two- and three-dimensional imaging. Ultrasound Obstet Gynecol 2005;25(5):473–7.
19. Platt LD, Santulli T Jr, Carlson DE, et al. Three-dimensional ultrasonography in obstetrics and gynecology: preliminary experience. Am J Obstet Gynecol 1998;178:1199–206.

The Utility of Volume Sonography for the Detection of Fetal Spine Abnormalities

Noam Lazebnik, MD[a,*], Eran Bornstein, MD[b],
Ilan E. Timor-Tritsch, MD, RDMS[b]

KEYWORDS

- Volume ultrasound
- Fetal spine abnormalities
- Technical principals

Sonographic evaluation of the fetal vertebral column is essential for fetal central nervous system evaluation and valuable for ruling out genetic conditions. The development of volume ultrasound in the early 1990s[1–4] led several groups to study the fetal skeleton using the maximum intensity projection (MIP) mode, also termed "maximum transparency" or the "X-ray" mode.[5–12] Johnson and coworkers[8] performed three-dimensional studies of the fetal spine on 28 fetuses (16 normal and 12 abnormal). Fifteen of the 16 normal fetal spines were visualized completely. In cases of neural tube defects, a three-dimensional approach was superior for identifying the specific vertebral level of the lesion and recognizing the presence of scoliosis. Pilu and colleagues,[13] however, determined that a normal three-dimensional evaluation of the bony spine is not always reassuring, and may miss small, subtle, and low localized spina bifida. Similarly to others, they did recognize the additive value of the three-dimensional scan for identifying the precise location of a spinal lesion using the twelfth rib as a marker for T12.[13,14]

This article provides an overview for obtaining and manipulating fetal vertebrae three-dimensional data to obtain the necessary diagnostic views. Additional technical information is provided elsewhere in this issue. This discussion is limited to include only the most common fetal vertebral abnormalities. The same technical principals, however, enable detection of many additional abnormalities.

PROPER TECHNIQUE

Both transabdominal and transvaginal studies are practical for volume acquisition depending on the orientation of the fetal spine and the fetal size. Acquisition is best performed along the median plane of the trunk with beam origin at the posterior of the fetus. The authors generally use a 30- to 40-degree angle sweep to include the entire fetus within a single frame. If acquisition is not performed within the median plane, the volume may be manipulated to obtain appropriate sagittal and coronal planes. MIP mode rendering facilitates detection of skeletal anomalies, such as hemivertebra, sacral agenesis, and agenesis of ribs, and enables evaluation of the three ossification centers of each vertebra.[14,15]

The three-dimensional approach is extremely useful for studying the spine, vertebrae, ribs, pelvic bones, and the spinal cord. Not only can one simultaneously visualize three orthogonal planes, but also scroll through the volume along any given orientation. Through this one may confirm the precise anatomic location of a vertebral abnormality, using known anatomic landmarks for reference. Another extremely important tool is the "marker dot." Typically, this dot is located at the

---

[a] Department of Obstetrics and Gynecology, Case Western Reserve University, University Hospitals of Cleveland, 11100 Euclid Avenue, Cleveland, OH 44106, USA
[b] New York University School of Medicine, 550 First Avenue, Room 9N26, New York, NY 10016, USA
* Corresponding author.
E-mail address: noam.lazebnik@uhhospitals.org (N. Lazebnik).

intersection of three orthogonal planes and is freely movable by the user to pinpoint a given structure on three planes simultaneously.

Fig. 1 demonstrates multiplanar images of the fetal spine with the "thick slice" rendering technique and MIP mode (**Fig. 1**D). In **Fig. 1**E a different color scheme was used to enhance further the fetal bony structures. **Fig. 2** demonstrates the fetal spine rendered using MIP mode, demonstrating the three processes of the vertebrae and the rib cage and iliac bones. It is important to note that the use of real-time three-dimensional, also known as four-dimensional, may be useful for performing the skeletal evaluation during fetal motion.

NEURAL TUBE DEFECTS

Neural tube defects occur if there is interference with physiologic closure of the neural tube around the 28th day postfertilization. The normal brain and

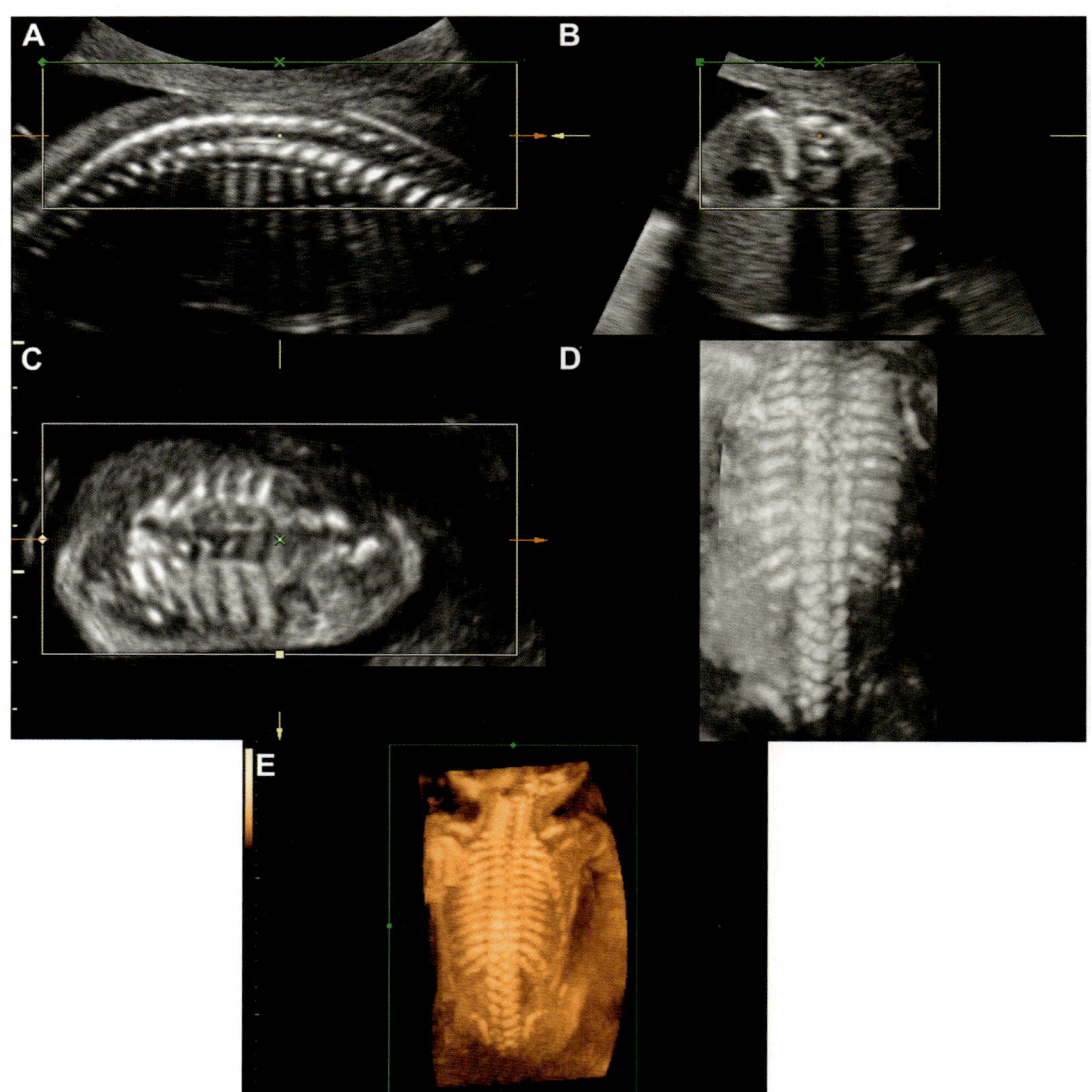

Fig. 1. Multiplanar display of the fetal spine with the sagittal plane (*A*) and axial plane (*B*) demonstrating the complete vertebrae and the coronal longitudinal plane (*C*). The "thick slice" technique was applied to obtain the rendered image in the MIP mode (*D*). Using this technique, the slice thickness can be adjusted, controlling the tissue width that is visualized by the final rendered image. (*E*) Rendered three-dimensional image of the fetal spine, vertebra, ribs, and the pelvic bones. The MIP mode and unique color scheme are used to document better the bony structures.

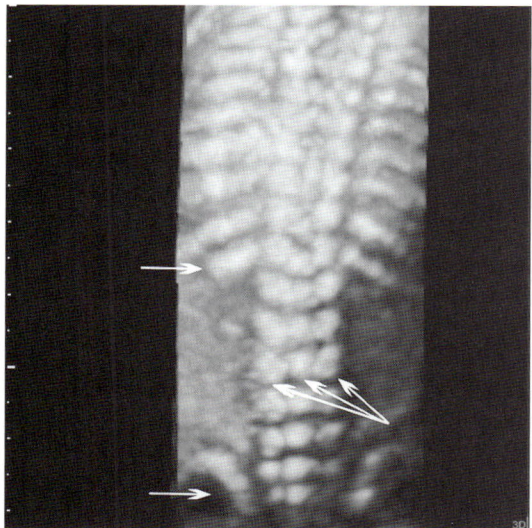

Fig. 2. The fetal spine rendered using MIP mode and demonstrating the three processes of each vertebra (the two lateral processes and the posterior process are marked with arrows). The rib cage can also be evaluated and assist in precise localization of vertebral defects. The twelfth rib is marked with an arrow and correlates with the level of T12. The iliac crests is also seen (*arrow*).

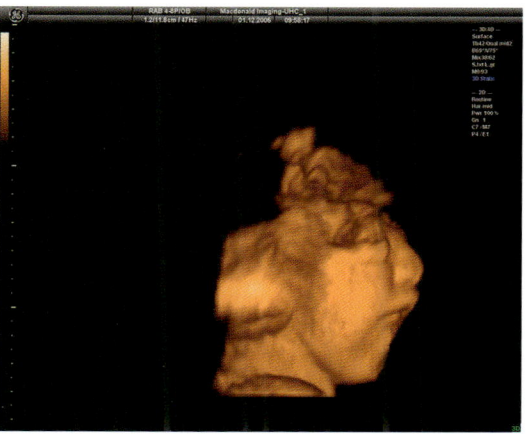

Fig. 3. Rendered three-dimensional image of the profile of an anencephalic fetus at 19 weeks. The entire frontal bone is missing and disorganized brain tissue is seen superior to the eyes.

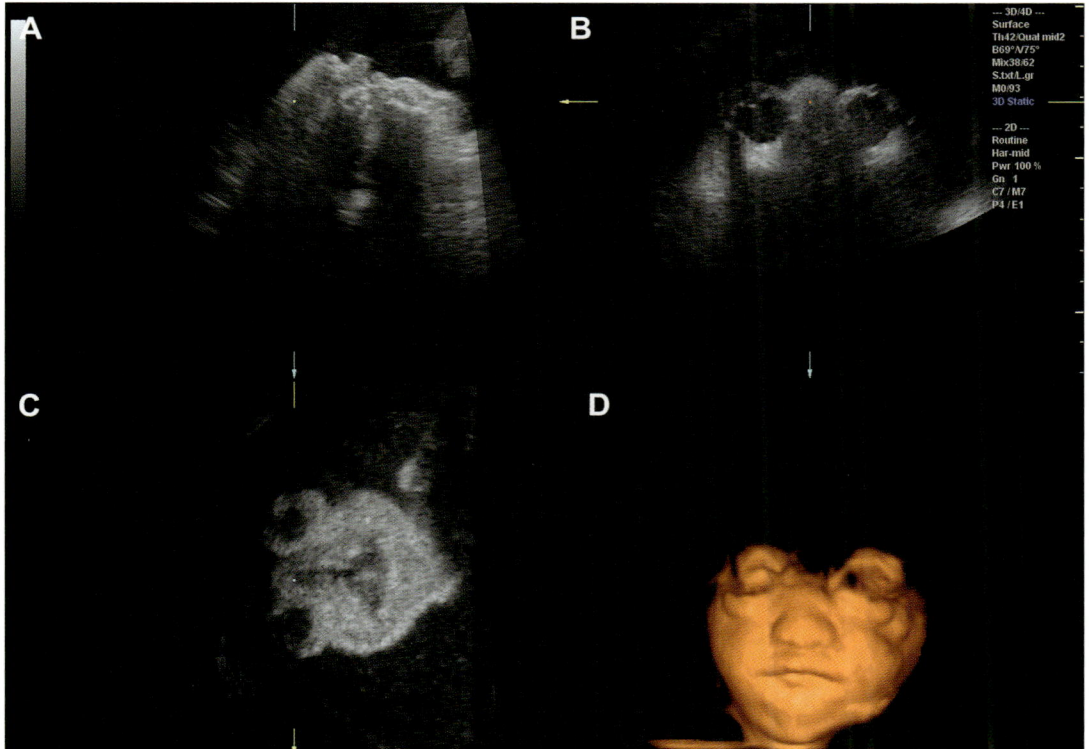

Fig. 4. The three orthogonal planes and a rendered three-dimensional image of the fetus seen in **Fig. 3**. The coronal image (*C*) demonstrates lack of calvarial bones.

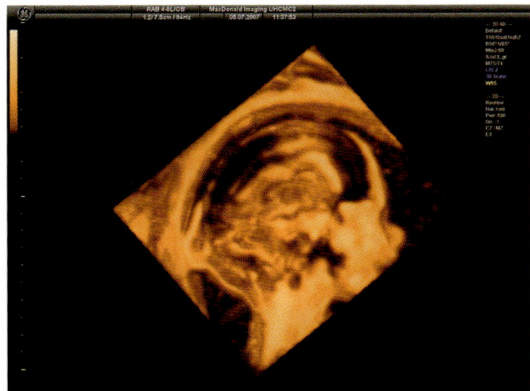

Fig. 5. Thin-sliced rendered three-dimensional image showing a posterior skull defect through which meninges and brain tissue herniated for this 20-week fetus with posterior encephalocele and final diagnosis of Walker-Warburg syndrome.

may affect the brain, spinal cord, and meninges. The severity of the abnormality differs between affected fetuses and the incidence of neural tube defects is approximately 1 to 3 per 1000 worldwide.

The spectrum of neural tube defects includes three types of defects: (1) anencephaly, (2) encephalocele, and (3) spina bifida.[16] The most severe form is anencephaly, which occurs when the "cephalic" or head end of the neural tube fails to close, resulting in absence of a major portion of the brain, skull, and scalp. Infants with this disorder are born without a forebrain and cerebrum. The remaining brain tissue is often exposed and not covered by bone or skin (**Figs. 3** and **4**).

Encephaloceles are rare neural tube defects characterized by sac-like protrusions of the brain and the membranes that cover it through openings in the skull. These defects are caused by failure of the neural tube to close completely during fetal development. The result is a groove down the midline of the upper part of the skull, the area between the forehead and nose, or the back of the skull (**Figs. 5** and **6**). Encephaloceles are often associated with neurologic problems and may be associated with known genetic conditions, such as Walker-Warburg syndrome. Usually,

spinal cord develop as a groove, which folds over to become a tube (the neural tube). Layers of tissues that normally emerge from this tube form the brain and spinal cord and their covering tissues, including parts of the spine and meninges. Failure of the neural tube to develop normally

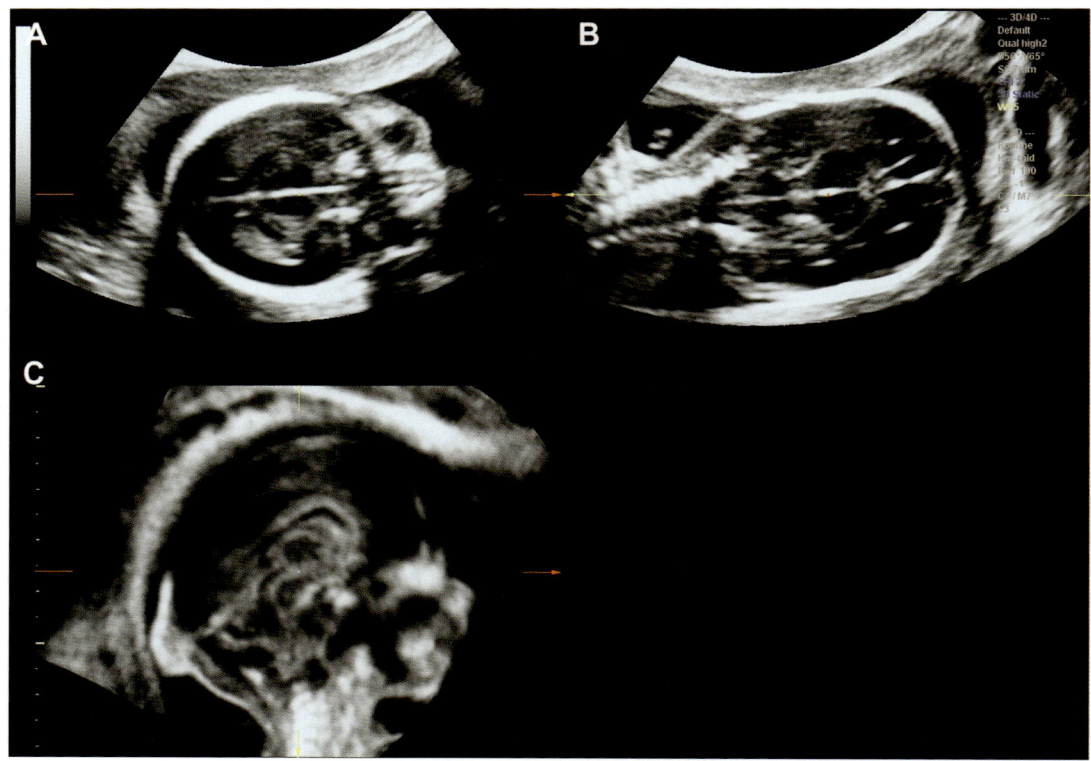

Fig. 6. The three orthogonal views and a rendered three-dimensional image of the fetus seen in **Fig. 5**. The encephalocele can be seen only on the coronal view.

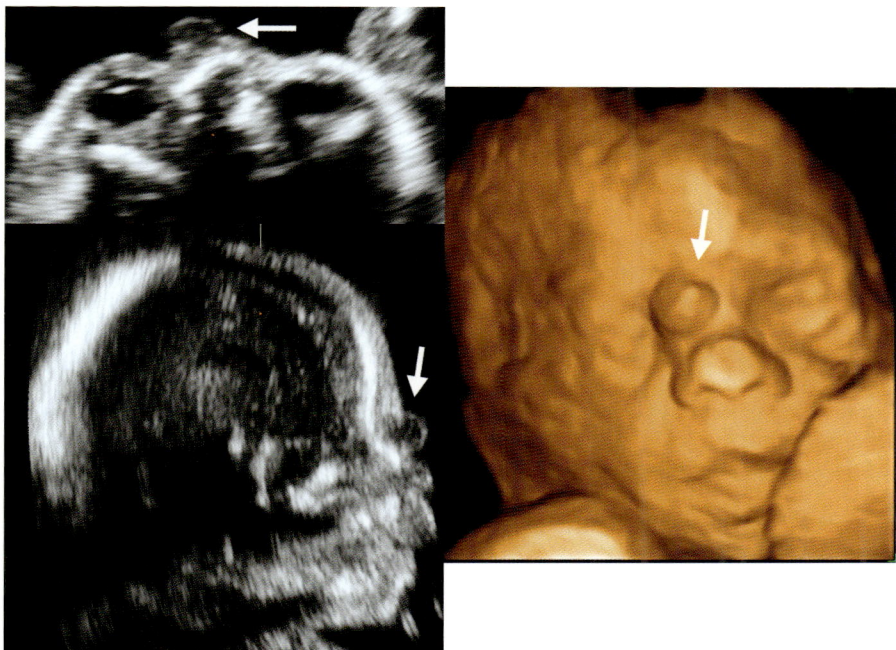

Fig. 7. A fetus with anterior encephalocele (*arrows*). The sagittal view shows the skull defect. Only the meninges are seen herniating out.

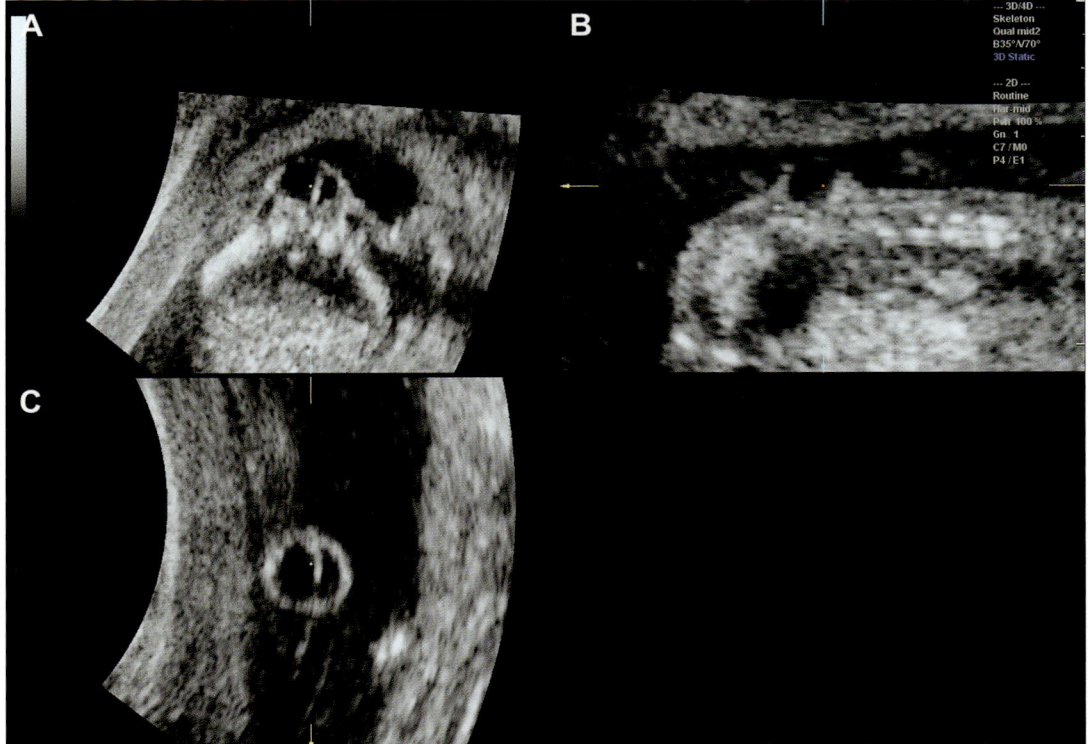

Fig. 8. A 22-week fetus with sacral open neural tube defect (meningocele). The anomaly in the axial (*A*), the sagittal (*B*), and the coronal planes (*C*) is clearly seen.

encephaloceles are dramatic deformities diagnosed in utero using an ultrasound study, but occasionally a small encephalocele in the nasal and forehead region is undetected (**Fig. 7**). Encephaloceles are often accompanied by craniofacial abnormalities or other brain malformations. Symptoms and associated abnormalities for encephaloceles may include hydrocephalus, spastic quadriplegia, microcephaly, ataxia, developmental delay, vision problems, mental and growth retardation, and seizures. There is a genetic component to the condition; it often occurs in families with a history of spina bifida and anencephaly in family members or might be a phenotypic expression of an unrelated genetic syndrome, such as Meckel-Gruber syndrome.

There are four types of spina bifida. They differ in severity and the tissue involved. Spina bifida occulta is the mildest and most common form in which one or more vertebrae are malformed. The name "occulta," which means "hidden," indicates that the malformation, or opening in the spine, is covered by a layer of skin. This form of spina bifida rarely causes disability or symptoms.

Closed neural tube defects make up the second type of spina bifida. These are a diverse group of defects in which the spinal cord is affected by a malformation of fat, bone, or membranes. In some patients there are few or no symptoms; in others the malformation causes incomplete paralysis with urinary and bowel dysfunction.

The third type of defect, meningocele, is characterized by the meninges protruding from the spinal opening. This malformation may or may not be covered by a layer of skin. Some patients with meningocele may have few or no symptoms, whereas others experience symptoms similar to those of closed neural tube defects.

Myelomeningocele, the fourth form, is the most severe and occurs when the spinal cord is exposed through the opening in the spine, resulting in partial or complete paralysis of the parts of the body below the level of the spinal opening. The paralysis may be so severe that the affected individual is unable to walk and may have urinary and bowel dysfunction.[16]

An example of a fetus with spina bifida detected at 22 weeks is demonstrated in **Figs. 8** and **9**. The

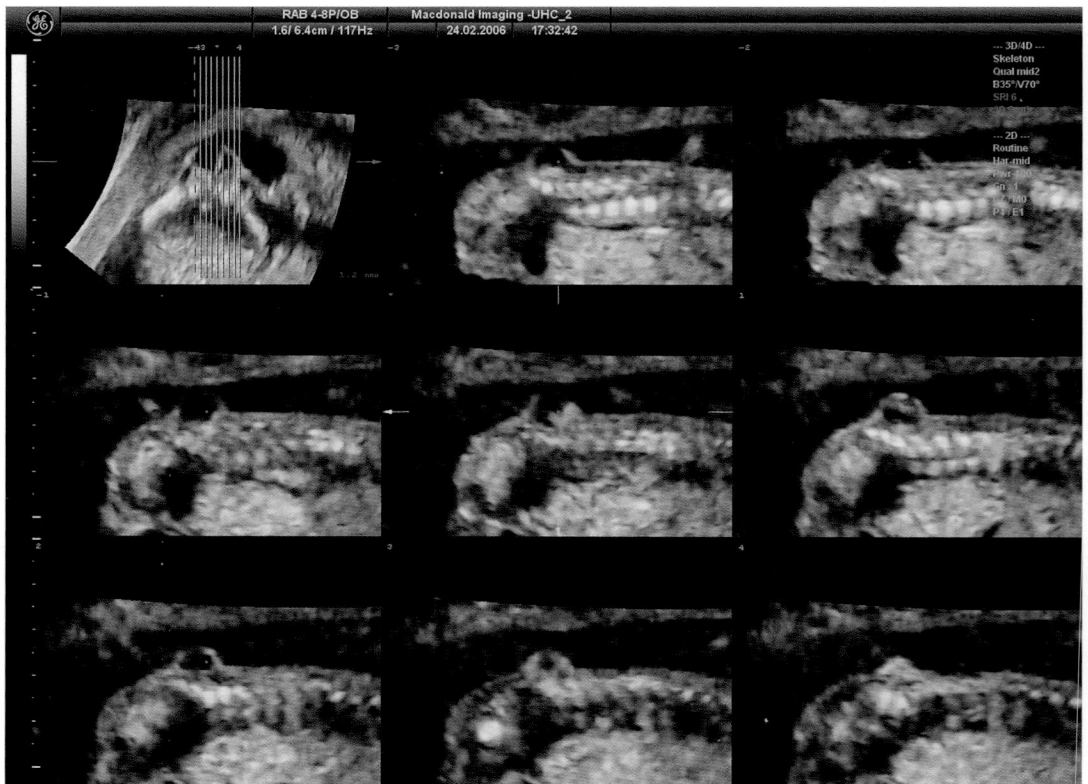

Fig. 9. Tomographic display mode demonstrating multiple successive sagittal views taken through the entire width of the spine defect. The lateral displacement of the cerebellar hemispheres can be evaluated at the different levels of the cerebellum. Only the meninges are herniating out.

sonographic volume was displayed in three orthogonal planes to visualize the anomaly in both the axial and the sagittal planes. Tomographic ultrasound imaging mode displays successive sagittal planes, improving delineation of extent of the anomaly and the nature of the tissue herniating through the defect to be meninges, suggesting meningocele. The vertebral column can be rendered using MIP mode for cases where the specific level of the spine defect cannot be determined easily using two-dimensional imaging and to illustrate the etiology of the herniating tissue (**Fig. 10**). Additionally, clinically significant open neural tube defects typically exhibit pathology of the posterior fossa (ie, the impacted cerebellum gives rise to the "banana sign," which is an indirect consequence of the vertebrae anomaly where the entire spinal cord is pulled downward) (**Fig. 11**).

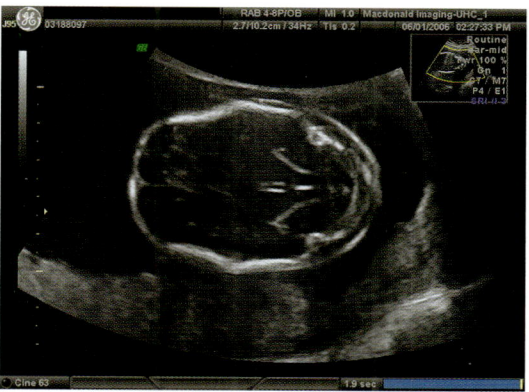

Fig. 11. The typical abnormalities associated with spinal open neural tube defect of the fetal skull (lemon sign) and the pulled down cerebellum (banana sign).

HEMIVERTEBRAE

The congenital vertebral anomalies are classified based on failure of formation; failure of segmentation; and a combination of the two (mixed).[17] The most common failure of formation anomaly is a hemivertebra. In this form, a portion of the vertebra is missing resulting in a small, triangular shaped "half vertebra" or hemivertebra. Congenital scoliosis is one type of structural spine deformation and hemivertebra is the most common anomaly causing congenital scoliosis (**Fig. 12**).[18] Hemivertebrae is associated with continued progression of scoliosis in extrauterine life.

Hemivertebrae may be isolated or may occur at multiple levels. It is frequently associated with other congenital anomalies.[18,19] These include other musculoskeletal anomalies, such as those of the spine, ribs, and limbs. Cardiac and genitourinary tract anomalies are the more common extramusculoskeletal anomalies seen with hemivertebrae. Anomalies of the central nervous system and gastrointestinal tract are also reported. Hemivertebra may be part of a syndrome including Jarcho–Levin, Klippel-Feil, and VACTERL association (Vertebral anomalies, Anal atresia, Cardiovascular anomalies, Tracheoesophageal fistula, Esophageal atresia, Renal [kidney] or radial anomalies, preaxial Limb anomalies).

Coronal display of the vertebral column facilitates easy visualization of the vertebral bodies including the three ossification centers and the ribs (**Fig. 13**). As with other skeletal anomalies, use of the MIP mode may assist in diagnosing this condition by demonstrating absence of part of the vertebra or one of its processes.

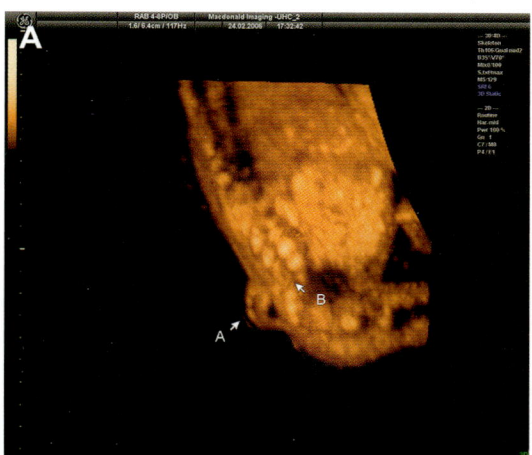

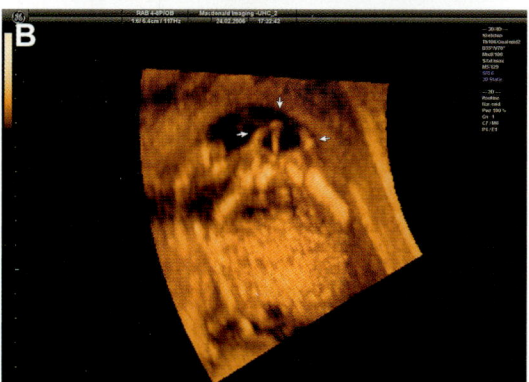

Fig. 10. The fetus seen in **Figs. 8** and **9**. The vertebral column can be rendered using MIP mode to demonstrate the spine defect (A) and to illustrate the nature of the tissue herniating out (B).

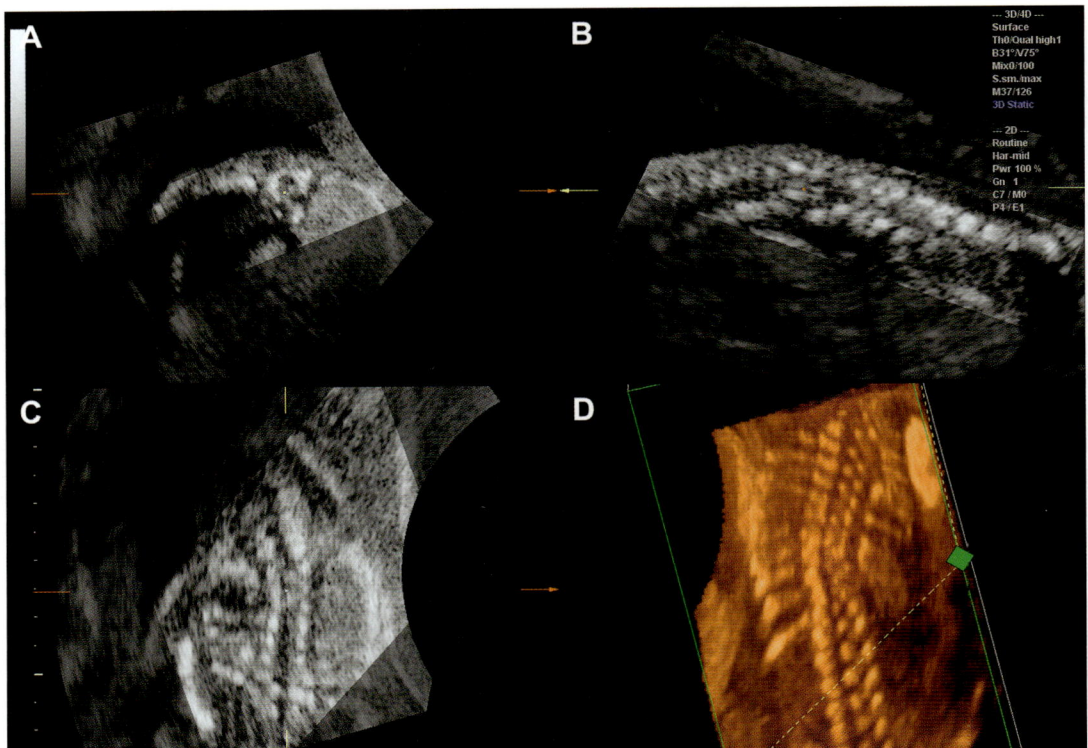

Fig. 12. A 23-week fetus diagnosed with VACTREL association. The spinal defect is clearly seen on the three orthogonal planes (A–C) and the three-dimensional rendered image (D) using MIP mode. Significant scoliosis also is seen.

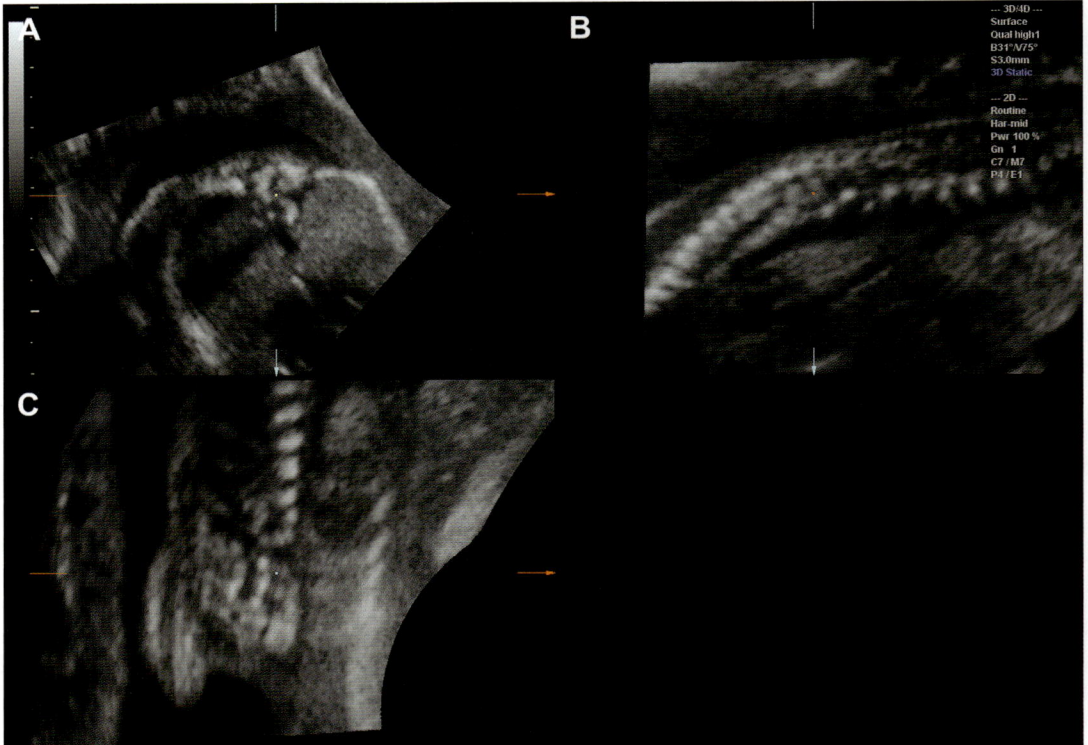

Fig. 13. The three orthogonal planes are used to show the failure of lateral vertebral formation resulting in a hemivertebra anomaly.

TETHERED SPINAL CORD OR OCCULT SPINAL DYSRAPHISM

Tethered spinal cord or occult spinal dysraphism is likely the result of improper growth of the neural tube during fetal development, and is closely linked to spina bifida. It is a rare neurologic disorder (occurring in 0.05–0.25 of 1000 births) and caused by tissue attachments that limit the movement of the spinal cord within the spinal column resulting in abnormal stretching of the spinal cord. Tethered spinal cord may go undiagnosed until adulthood, when sensory and motor problems and loss of bowel and bladder control emerge. The delayed presentation of symptoms is related to the degree of strain placed on the spinal cord over time. In children, symptoms may include lesions, hairy patches, dimples, or fatty tumor on the lower back; foot and spinal deformities; weakness in the legs; low back pain; scoliosis; and incontinence.[20]

Closed spinal defects, such as "subtle skin-covered spinal dysraphism," are difficult to detect in utero by a routine two-dimensional ultrasound study. This group of anomalies includes a tethered cord (tight filum terminale syndrome); diastematomyelia; subcutaneous or interspinal lipoma; and epidermoid and dermoid cysts.

During normal fetal development, the conus medullaris (CM), which is situated at the sacral region of the vertebral column, ascends to its final location at birth. Review of the literature demonstrates a limited number of studies focused on the CM. Wilson and Prince[21] used MR imaging to determine the anatomic location of the normal CM throughout childhood and demonstrated it is proximal to the L2 vertebra. Robbin and colleagues[22] studied the fetal CM using two-dimensional ultrasound techniques. In a recent study by Zalel and colleagues,[23] the researchers describe the normal location of the CM and determined the timeline of its ascent during human gestation using two-dimensional imaging. To locate the CM precisely, they obtained sagittal and coronal longitudinal views identifying known anatomic landmarks. The upper pole of the kidney was considered the T11 vertebra, and the lower rib was T12. Verification was done by counting the vertebra from the lumbosacral junction upward. Zalel and colleagues[23] concluded that the CM could be

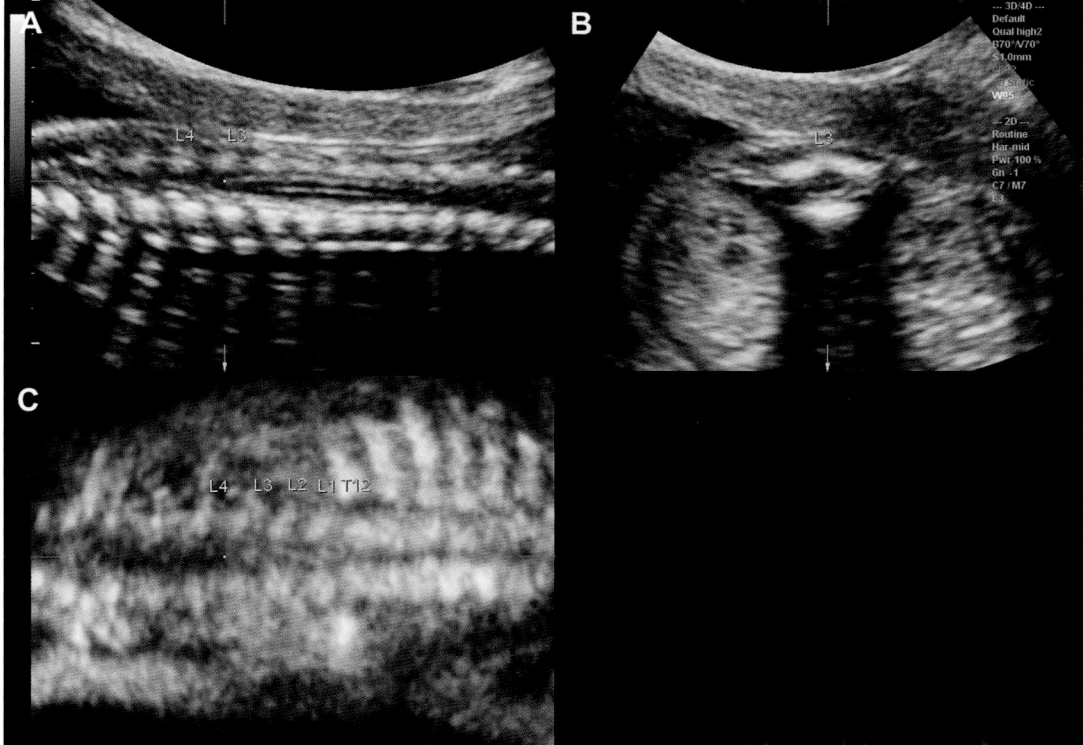

Fig. 14. A 36-week fetus. The sagittal plane demonstrates the distal end of the CM (*A*). The other two planes (*B, C*) confirm the location by using the coronal plan to identify the twelfth rib/T12 and count the vertebra caudally. The marker dot identifies the location of the distal end of the CM on all three planes.

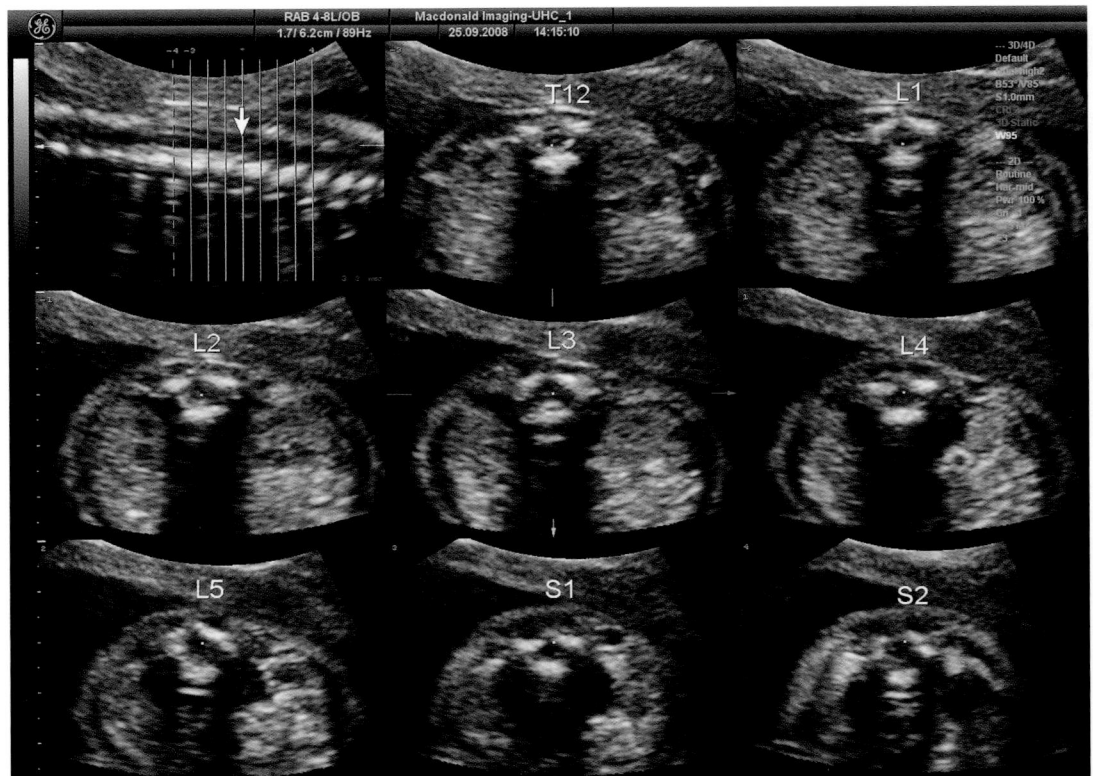

Fig. 15. The tomographic display mode is used to verify that neural tissue is not seen distal to L4. The marker dot identifies the location of the distal end of the CM on all tomographic slices.

sonographically identified and followed throughout pregnancy and a significant ascent of the CM was detected between 13 and 40 postmenstrual weeks from the level of L4 or more caudally, between 13 and 18 postmenstrual weeks of pregnancy, to the level of L1 to L2 at approximately 40 weeks. They also suggested that in fetuses whose CM termination levels are equivocal (L3) or abnormal (lower than L3–L4), a follow-up ultrasound study and additional work-up are indicated in early life.

Figs. 14 and 15 demonstrate the CM of a 36-week fetus suspected of having tethered spinal cord. The CM is seen lower than expected between L3 to L4. The use of the three orthogonal planes and the tomographic display mode enabled precise localization of the CM to be equivocal (L3–L4) late in gestation. The diagnosis was confirmed at 6 months of age.

SUMMARY

Volumetric sonography is extremely useful for examining the fetal spine, individual vertebrae, pelvic bones, and the spinal cord. By scrolling through the volume one may confirm the exact location of a vertebral abnormality using known anatomic landmarks as a reference point. The preferred three-dimensional rendering mode of the vertebral column is the MIP mode, which provides valuable information complementary to a conventional two-dimensional examination.

REFERENCES

1. Mueller GM, Weiner CP, Yankowitz J. Three-dimensional ultrasound in the evaluation of fetal head and spinal anomalies. Obstet Gynecol 1996;88: 372–8.
2. International Society of Ultrasound in Obstetrics & Gynecology Education Committee. Sonographic examination of the fetal central nervous system: guidelines for performing the basic examination and the fetal neurosonogram. Ultrasound Obstet Gynecol 2007;29(1):109–16.
3. Merz E, Bahlmann F, Weber G, et al. Three-dimensional ultrasonography in prenatal diagnosis. J Perinat Med 1995;23(3):213–22.
4. Steiner H, Spitzer D, Weiss-Wichert PH, et al. Three-dimensional ultrasound in prenatal diagnosis of skeletal dysplasia. Prenat Diagn 1995;15:373–7.

5. Platt LD, Santuli T Jr, Carlson DE, et al. Three-dimensional ultrasonography in obstetrics and gynecology: preliminary experience. Am J Obstet Gynecol 1998;178:1199–206.
6. Nelson TR, Pretorius DH. Visualization of the fetal thoracic skeleton with three-dimensional sonography: a preliminary report. Am J Roentgenol 1995; 164:1485–8.
7. Riccabona M, Johnson D, Pretorius DH, et al. Three dimensional ultrasound: display modalities in the fetal spine and thorax. Eur J Radiol 1996;22:141–5.
8. Johnson DD, Pretorius DH, Riccabona M, et al. Three-dimensional ultrasound of the fetal spine. Obstet Gynecol 1997;89:434–8.
9. Schild RL, Wallny T, Fimmers R, et al. Fetal lumbar spine volumetry by three-dimensional ultrasound. Ultrasound Obstet Gynecol 1999;13:335–9.
10. Ulm MR, Kratochwil A, Oberhuemer U, et al. Ultrasound evaluation of fetal spine length between 14 and 24 weeks of gestation. Prenat Diagn 1999;19:637–41.
11. Garjian KV, Pretorius DH, Budorick NE, et al. Fetal skeletal dysplasia: three-dimensional US: Initial experience. Radiology 2000;214:717–23.
12. Lee W, Chaiworapongsa T, Romero R, et al. A diagnostic approach for the evaluation of spina bifida by three-dimensional ultrasonography. J Ultrasound Med 2002;21(6):619–26.
13. Pilu G, Ghi T, Carletti A, et al. Three-dimensional ultrasound examination of the fetal central nervous system. Ultrasound Obstet Gynecol 2007;30(2): 233–45.
14. Esser T, Rogalla P, Sarioglu N, et al. Three-dimensional ultrasonographic demonstration of agenesis of the 12th rib in a fetus with trisomy 21. Ultrasound Obstet Gynecol 2006;27(6):714–5.
15. Kalache KD, Bamberg C, Proquitté H, et al. Three-dimensional multi-slice view: new prospects for evaluation of congenital anomalies in the fetus. J Ultrasound Med 2006;25(8):1041–9.
16. National Institute of Neurological Disorders and Stroke. Spina bifida fact sheet. Available at: http://www.ninds.nih.gov/disorders/spina_bifida/detail_spina_bifida.htm. Accessed November 7, 2008.
17. Erol B, Kusumi K, Lou B, et al. Etiology of congenital scoliosis. UPOJ 2002;15:37–42.
18. McMaster MJ, David CV. Hemivertebra as a cause of scoliosis. J Bone Joint Surg Br 1986;68:588–95.
19. Connor JM, Conner AN, Connor RAC, et al. Genetic aspects of early childhood scoliosis. Am J Med Genet 1987;27:419–24.
20. National Institute of Neurological Disorders and Stroke. NINDS tethered spinal cord syndrome information page. Available at: http://www.ninds.nih.gov/disorders/tethered_cord/tethered_cord.htm. Accessed November 7, 2008.
21. Wilson DA, Prince JR. MR imaging determination of the location of the normal conus medullaris throughout childhood. AJR Am J Roentgenol 1989;152: 1029–32.
22. Robbin ML, Filly RA, Goldstein RB. The normal location of the fetal conus medullaris. J Ultrasound Med 1994;13:541–6.
23. Zalel Y, Lehavi O, Aizenstein O, et al. Development of the fetal spinal cord: time of ascendance of the normal conus medullaris as detected by sonography. J Ultrasound Med 2006;25(11):1397–401.

Fetal Neuroimaging of Neural Migration Disorder

Ritsuko K. Pooh, MD, PhD

KEYWORDS

- Fetus • Prenatal • Neuroimaging • Migration disorder
- Lissencephaly • Cortical development

Many brain malformations are closely related to neuronal migration disorders.[1] Neuronal migration disorders include focal cerebrocortical dysgenesis, heterotopia, polymicrogyria, lissencephaly or pachygyria, and schizencephaly. These disorders are caused by the abnormal migration of neurons in the developing brain and nervous system. Neurons must migrate from their origin areas to their final anatomic location within the central nervous system (CNS) where they must settle into proper neural circuits. Neuronal migration, which occurs as early as the second month of gestation, is controlled by a complex assortment of chemical guides and signals. When these signals are absent or incorrect, neurons do not migrate appropriately.

Fetal neuroimaging, through advances in ultrasound and MR imaging, has contributed to the field of fetal medicine in prenatal detection of many congenital CNS anomalies, such as prosencephalic disorders, neurulation disorders, intracranial tumors, cysts, and brain damage attributable to intrauterine insults. In addition, prenatal imaging assessment of the fetal CNS contributes to more effective prenatal/postnatal management. Although migration disorders occur during early gestational stage, their phenotypic expression appears in late pregnancy, when sonographic assessment of the cortical development is difficult because of fetal cranial ossification. Antenatal cortical assessment is, at present, one of the most challenging fields of fetal medicine.

NORMAL CORTICAL DEVELOPMENT

Neuronal migration occurs between 3 and 5 months' gestation. In early brain development, nerve cells migrate to their final anatomic destinations to populate and form the six layers of the cerebral cortex. When the brain first forms, neurons are generated in a region of the ventricular zone and "crawl" to the cortical surface. There are two modes of cell migration: tangential migration and radial migration.[2] The first and earlier mechanism is movement by translocation of the cell body.[3] This movement results in the prepalate formation. The second mechanism is radial migration, in which migrating cells are generated by the radial glial progenitors. Travel instructions and guides are served to migrating cells and are controlled by complicated molecular machinery.

Owing to recent advanced sonographic technology and fast MR technology, detailed morphologic structures of the fetal brain are detectable as early as the late first and early second trimesters. Phenotypic expression of migration disorders appears in late pregnancy and therefore seems difficult to detect by the end of the second trimester. During pregnancy, one of the most comprehensive imaging planes for evaluation of fetal cortical development is the anterior coronal section, in which the bilateral sylvian fissures are well demonstrated, as shown in **Fig. 1**. This plane is acquired sonographically by way of the anterior fontanelle window. During the latter half of the second trimester, the cortical structure macroscopically develops. The most distinct morphologic alteration seems to affect the structure of the sylvian fissure between approximately 20 and 30 weeks. The sylvian fissure is thus one of the morphologic landmarks indicating cortical development through normal neuronal migration. Developmental delay of the sylvian fissures

CRIFM Clinical Research Institute of Fetal Medicine PMC, 3-7, Uehommachi, Tennoji, Osaka #543-0001, Japan
E-mail address: rkpooh@guitar.ocn.ne.jp

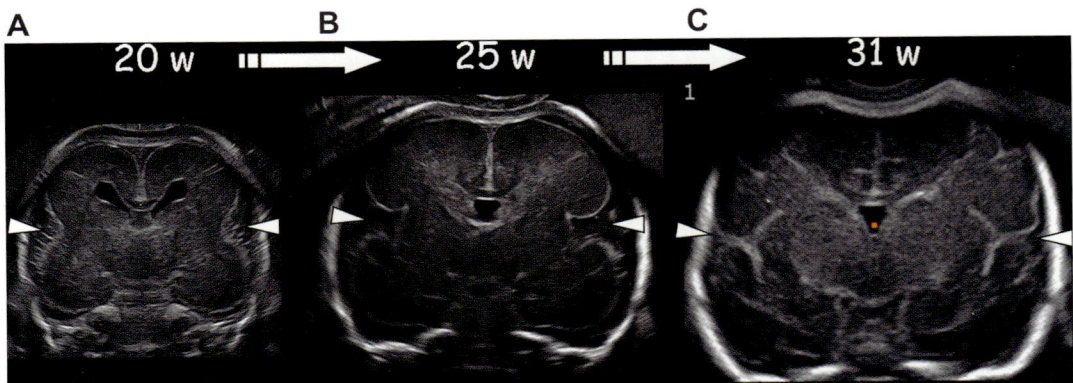

Fig. 1. Changing appearance of sylvian fissure in the anterior coronal section by transvaginal sonography. At 20 weeks of gestation, the bilateral sylvian fissures (*arrowheads*) appear as indentations (*left, A*). With cortical development, sylvian fissures are formed during the latter half of the second trimester (*middle, B*) and become the lateral sulci (*right, C*). Sylvian fissure appearance is one of the most reliable ultrasound markers for the assessment of cortical development.

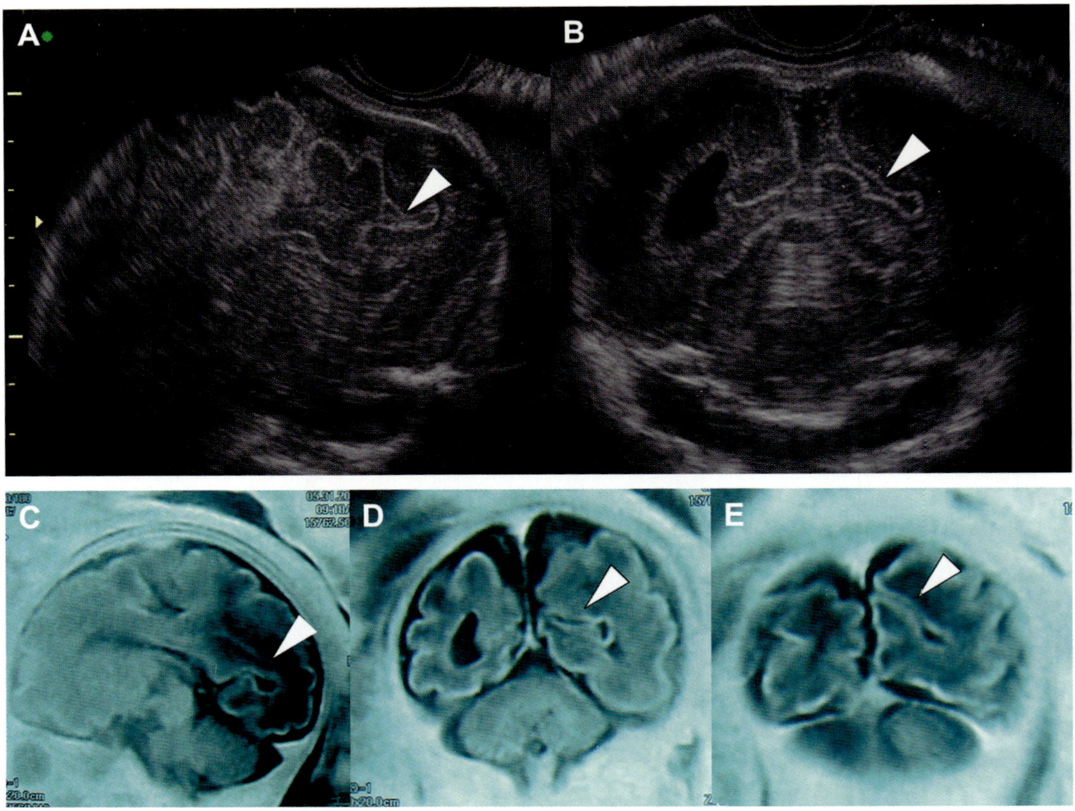

Fig. 2. Abnormal sulcal formation at 31 weeks and 5 days of gestation. (*Upper*) Transvaginal ultrasound images. Sagittal (*left, A*) and posterior coronal (*right, B*) sections. Arrowheads indicate abnormal sulcal formation. (*Lower*) MR images for the same gestation. Same findings as shown by sonography were confirmed by the sagittal (*left, C*) and posterior coronal (*middle, right, D, E*) sections.

during the second and third trimesters should bring suspicion for migration disorder.

MIGRATION DISORDERS

Migration disorder can result in structurally abnormal or missing areas of the brain in the cerebral hemispheres, cerebellum, brainstem, or hippocampus. Disorders of neuronal migration, in order of increasing severity, include focal cerebrocortical dysgenesis, heterotopia, polymicrogyria, lissencephaly or pachygyria, and schizencephaly.

In migrational disorders, hypoplasia or agenesis of the corpus callosum often accompanies gyral abnormality.[2] The causes of disorders of migration are varied and include environmental toxic conditions or genetic metabolic disorders.

Detection of polymicrogyria as early as 24 weeks has been reported[4] but more commonly prenatal sonographic suspicions for migration disorder arise during the third trimester.

FOCAL CEREBROCORTICAL DYSGENESIS

Migration disorders associated with cerebrocortical dysgenesis may occur anywhere intracranially. The prognosis varies with the specific disorder, degree of brain abnormality, and subsequent neurologic deficiencies. Occasionally minor gyral/sulcal abnormality is detectable using ultrasound study of the fetal brain as shown in **Figs. 2** and **3**. **Figs. 4** and **5** demonstrate unilateral maldevelopment at 20 weeks' gestation as detected by ultrasonography and MR imaging because of unilateral hemispheric migration disorder of the brain. Histologic findings subsequent to termination of pregnancy showed the distinct differences in brain structure between the right and left hemispheres (see **Fig. 5**). **Figs. 6** and **7** demonstrate asymmetric development of the ventricular zone and cortical structure between hemispheres. Postnatal multiple heterotopias were confirmed by MR imaging along with intractable convulsions.

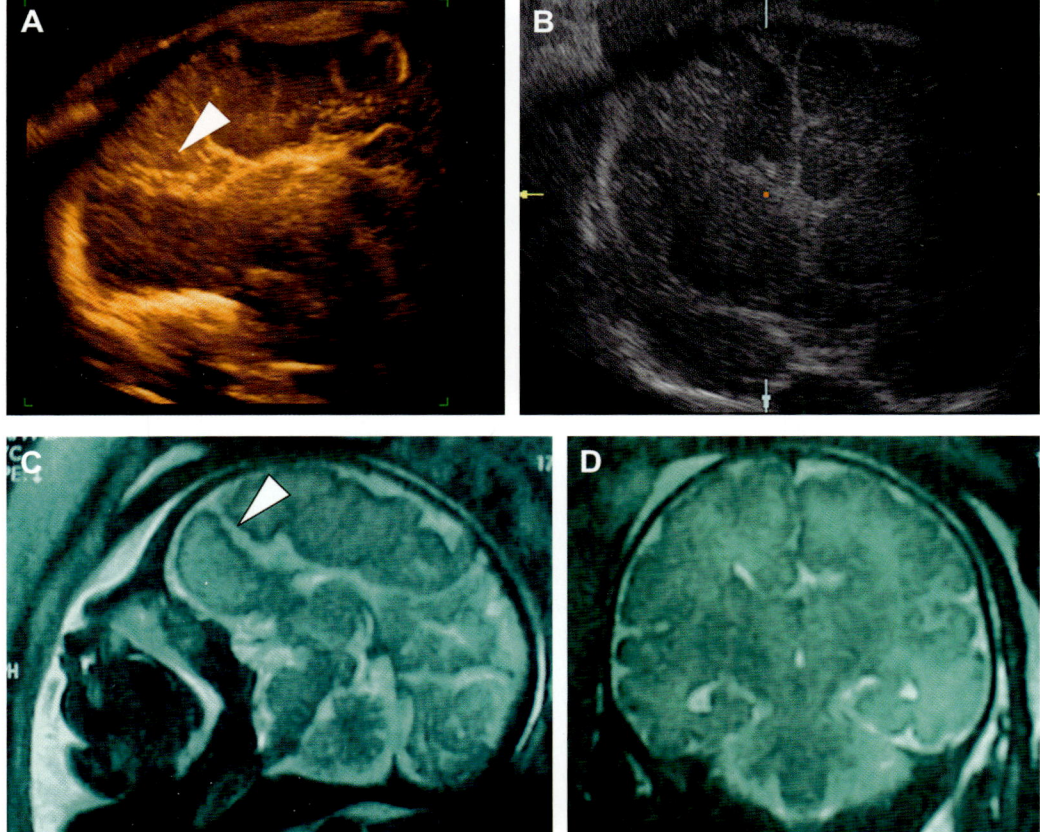

Fig. 3. Abnormal sulcal formation with agenesis of the corpus callosum at 36 weeks of gestation. Transvaginal ultrasound images. Sagittal (*upper left, A*) and anterior coronal (*upper right, B*) sections. No corpus callosum is seen. Arrowhead indicates abnormal sulcal formation. MR images for the same gestation. Same findings as shown by sonography were confirmed by the sagittal (*lower left, C*) and anterior coronal (*lower right, D*) sections.

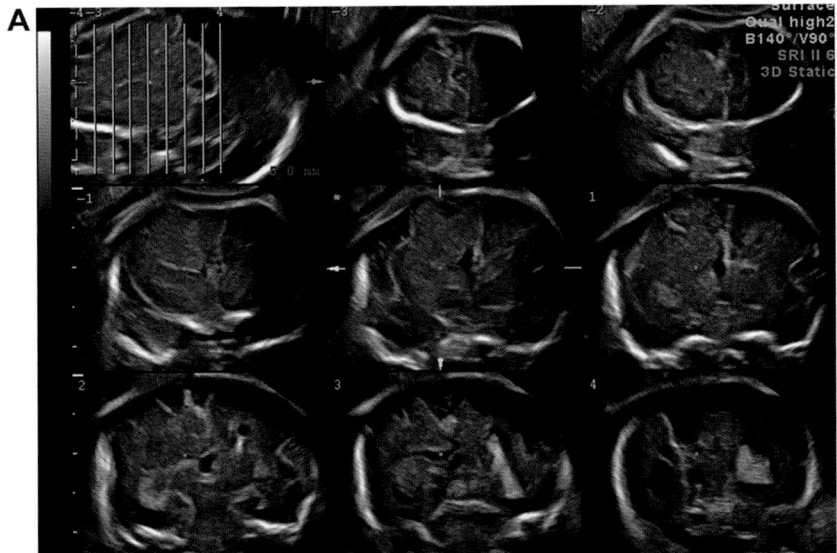

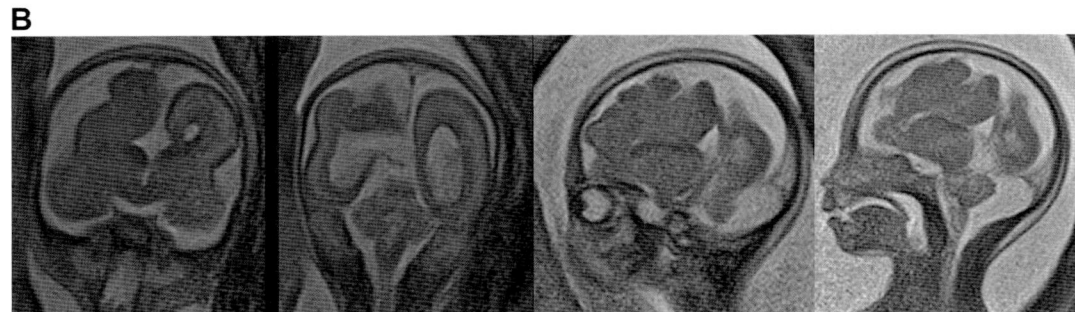

Fig. 4. Migration disorder of unilateral hemisphere at 18 weeks of gestation. (*upper six images, A*) Tomographic coronal image of the brain. Note the markedly different appearance of the bilateral hemispheres. (*Lower four images, B*) MR images of the same gestational age. Anterior-coronal, posterior-coronal, parasagittal and mid-sagittal sections (left to right). Unilateral abnormal brain development was caused by the migration disorder.

LISSENCEPHALY

Lissencephaly is characterized by lack of gyral development. Previously lissencephaly was classified into two types. In type I the surface of the brain is smooth, whereas in type II the surface demonstrates a cobblestone appearance. A recent classification is based on associated malformations and genetic causes.[5] Five major groups of lissencephaly are recognized: (1) Classic lissencephaly (previously known as type 1 lissencephaly), including lissencephaly due to the LIS1 gene mutation, which subdivides into type 1 isolated lissencephaly and the Miller-Dieker syndrome, lissencephaly due to the doublecortin (DCX) gene mutation, (2) X-linked lissencephaly with agenesis of the corpus callosum, linked to the ARX gene, (3) lissencephaly with cerebellar hypoplasia, including the Norman-Roberts syndrome linked to mutation in the reelin gene, (4) micro-lissencephaly (lissencephaly and microcephaly), and (5) cobblestone lissencephaly, including the Walker-Warburg syndrome, also known as HARD ± E syndrome (*h*ydrocephalus, *a*gyria, *r*etinal *d*ysplasia, with or without encephalocele), Fukuyama syndrome, and muscle-eye-brain (MEB) disease.

Several reports of prenatal diagnosis of lissencephaly are available.[6–8] **Fig. 8** shows the lissencephalic brain with abnormal brain circulation due to chromosomal aberration at 29 weeks and demonstrates bilateral shallow sylvian fissures, premature brain structure, and mild ventriculomegaly. Pachygyria in the third trimester from unknown cause is shown in **Fig. 9**. Classic

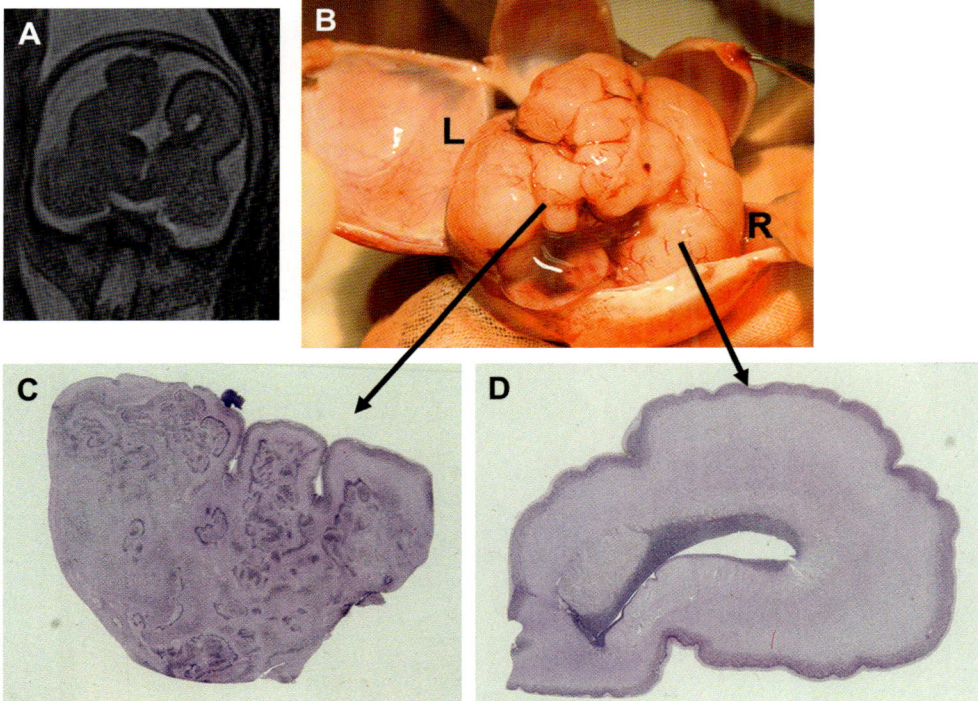

Fig. 5. Specimen from aborted fetus at 21 weeks of gestation and histologic findings (the same case as **Fig. 4**). (*Left upper, A*) Prenatal MR imaging, coronal section. (*Right upper, B*) Macroscopic intracranial finding at autopsy. (*Left lower, C*) Maldevelopment of the other hemisphere due to the migration disorder. (*Right lower, D*) Normal cerebral structure of normal hemisphere.

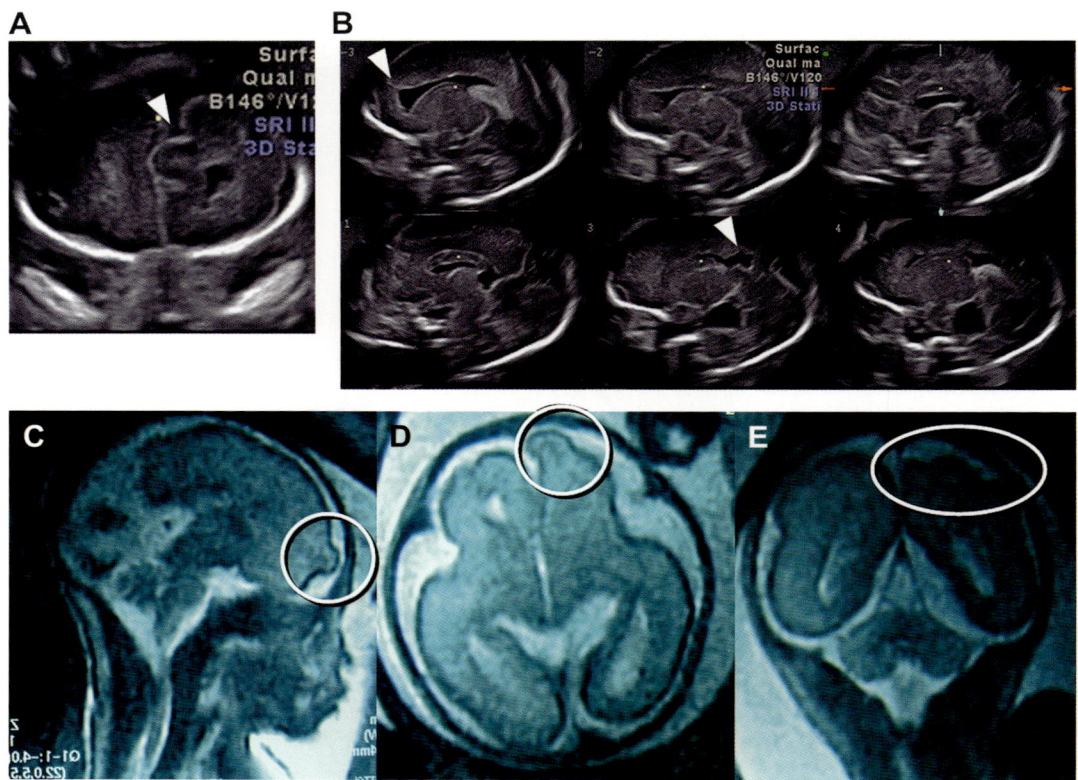

Fig. 6. Ultrasound and MR imaging of migration disorder at 25 weeks of gestation. (*Upper left, A*) Ultrasound anterior coronal section. Abnormal gyri and sulcus (*arrowhead*) are seen in the unilateral hemisphere. (*Upper right, B*) Tomographic ultrasound imaging, sagittal section. Abnormally asymmetrical shape of the ventricles (*arrowheads*) is demonstrated. (*Lower*) Fetal MR imaging at the same gestational age. In the sagittal (*left, C*) and axial (*middle, D*) sections, abnormal protrusion of the unilateral anterior lobe (*circle*) is seen. In the posterior coronal section (*right, E*), abnormal gyral formation (*oval*) is seen.

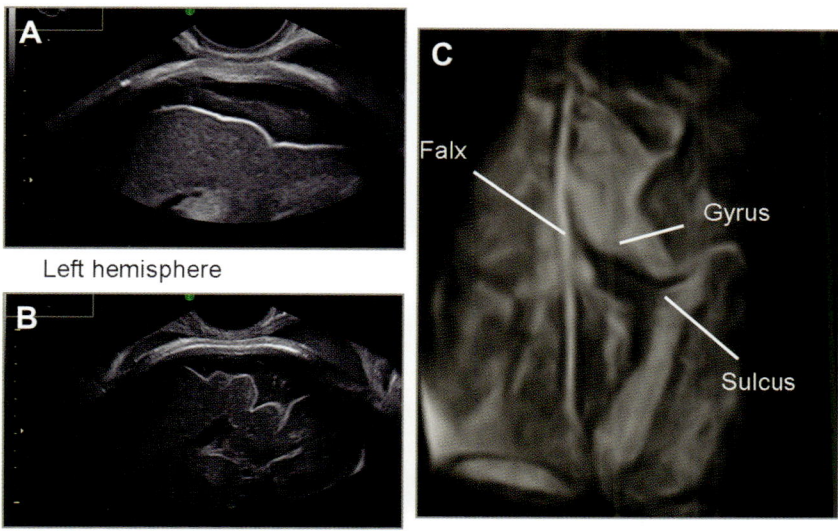

Fig. 7. Ultrasound imaging of abnormal cortical formation at 29 weeks of gestation. (the same case as **Fig. 6**). Parasagittal ultrasound image of the surface of left hemisphere (*upper left, A*) and right hemisphere (*lower left, B*). Note the marked difference in cortical formation between hemispheres. The right figure (*C*) demonstrates the surface anatomy of hemispheres by 3D ultrasound in parietal view. The different formation of gyrus and sulcus between hemispheres is clearly demonstrated.

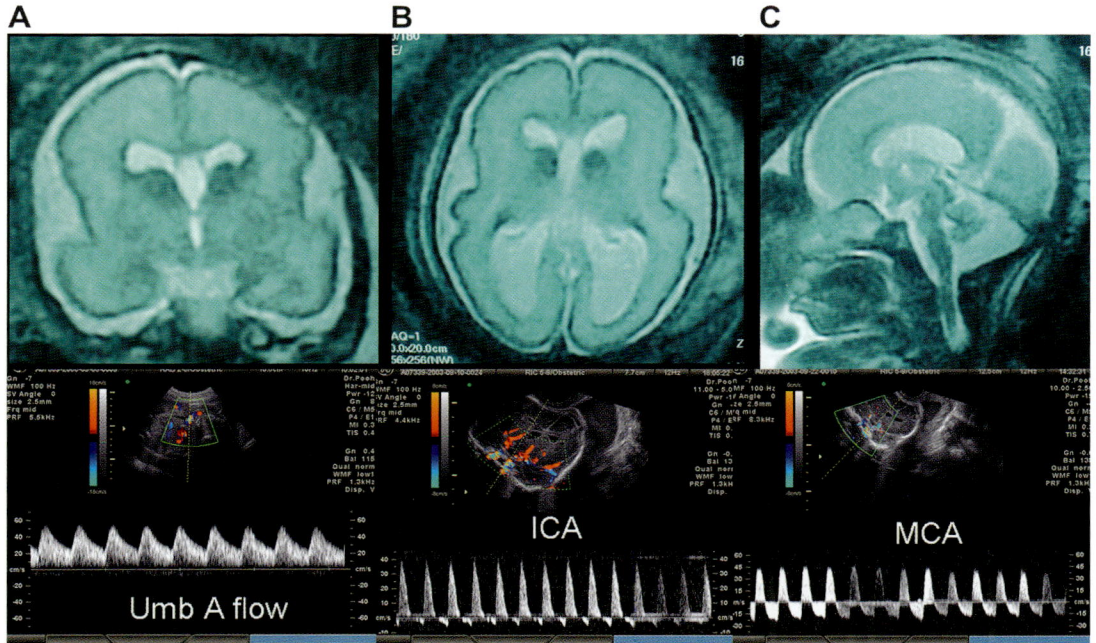

Fig. 8. Lissencephalic brain with abnormal brain circulation due to chromosomal aberration at 29 weeks. (*Upper*) Fetal MR images. Coronal, axial and mid-sagittal sections from left, (*A–C*). In coronal and axial sections, shallow sylvian fissures, premature brain structure, and mild ventriculomegaly are demonstrated. (*Lower*) Fetal blood flow waveforms. Umbilical artery flow is normal (*left, A*), but internal carotid artery (ICA, *B*) and middle cerebral artery (MCA, *C*) demonstrate reverse end-diastolic flow.

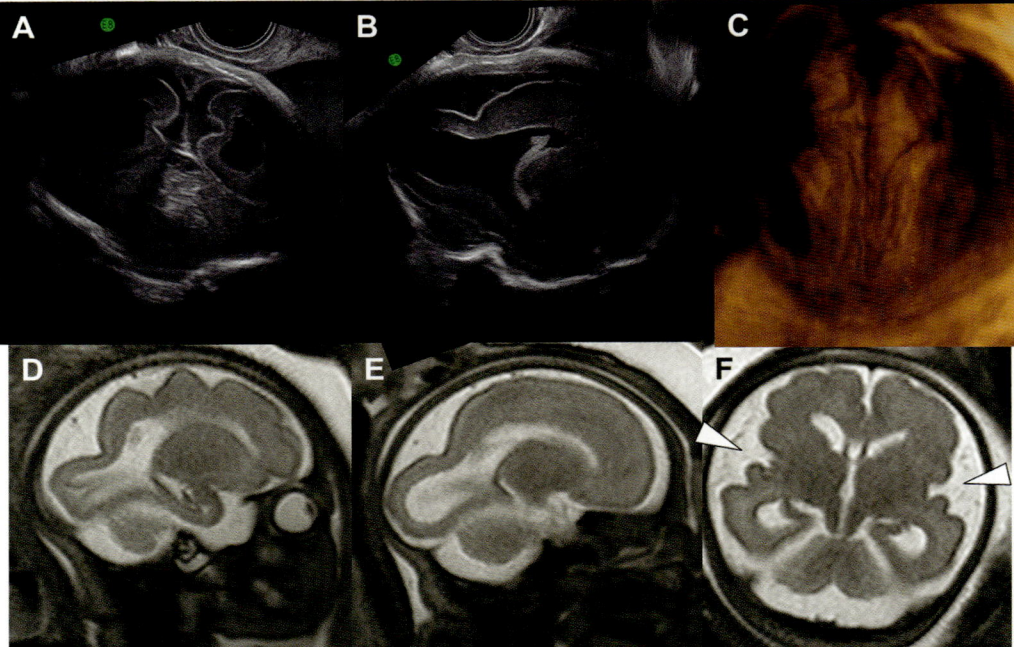

Fig. 9. Lissencephaly (pachygyria) at 33 weeks of gestation. (*Upper*) Transvaginal ultrasound pictures. Posterior coronal (*left*, A) and parasagittal (*middle*, B) sections show the smooth surface of the cerebral hemispheres. (*Upper right*, C) Surface anatomy of the cerebral superficial structure by 3D ultrasound in parietal view. (*Lower*) MR images for the same gestation. Parasagittal sections (*lower left and middle*, D, E) shows pachygyria. Anterior coronal section (*lower right*, F) demonstrates bilateral shallow sylvian fissures (*arrowheads*) with wide subarachnoid space around the hemispheres.

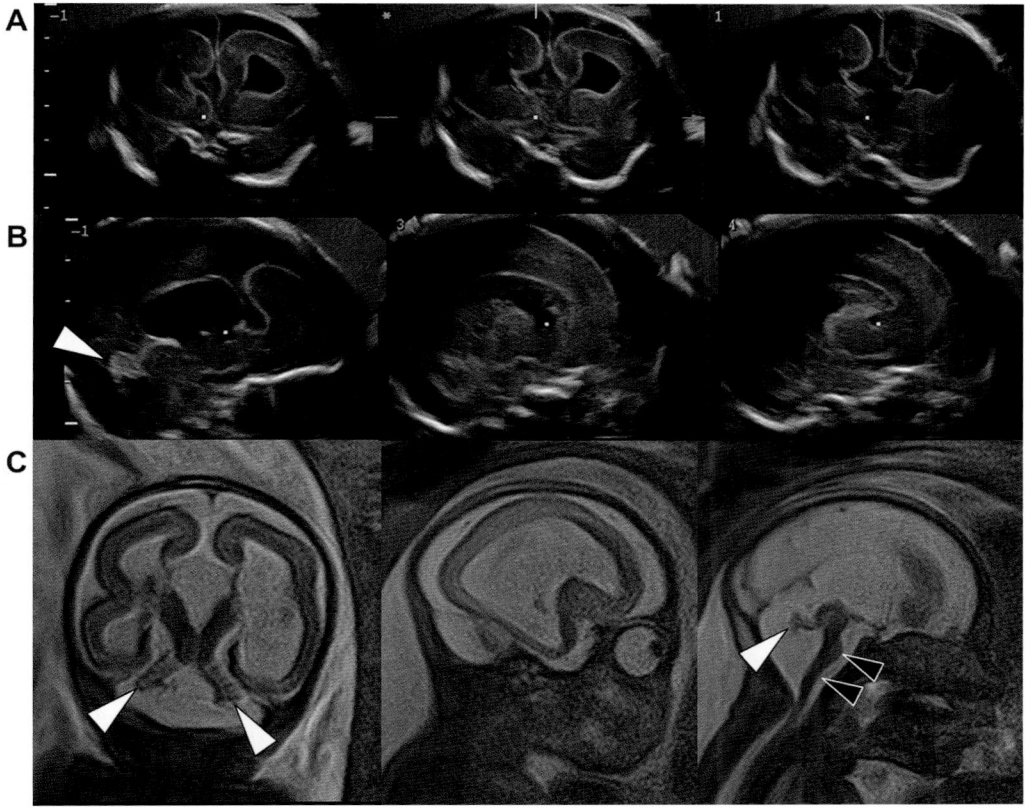

Fig. 10. Classical lissencephaly (type I lissencephaly) at 31 weeks of gestation. (*Upper three images, A*) Coronal tomographic ultrasound images. Note the smooth premature appearance of the bilateral hemispheres with ventriculomegaly. (*Middle three images, B*) Sagittal tomographic ultrasound images. Small cerebellum (*white arrowhead*) and smooth cerebri are demonstrated. (*Lower three images, C*) MR image for the same gestation. Coronal, parasagittal and mid-sagittal sections (left to right). The brain appearance is similar to that of a 10- to 12-week-brain. The cerebellar hemispheres also appear premature (*white arrowheads*). Prematurity of the brainstem (*black arrowheads*) may predict postnatal respiratory difficulty.

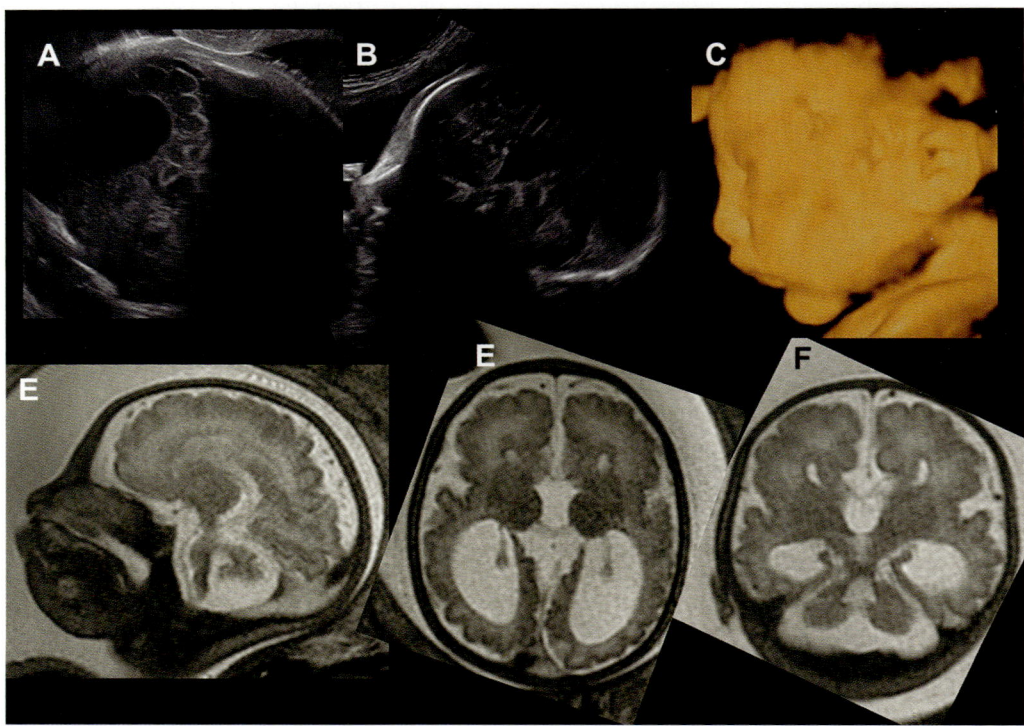

Fig. 11. Cobblestone lissencephaly (classical type II lissencephaly) with agenesis of the corpus callosum and cerebellar hypoplasia at 36 weeks of gestation. (*Upper*) Sonographic pictures of the posterior coronal (*left, A*) and midsagittal (*middle, B*) sections. Abnormal gyral formation is demonstrated. (*Upper right, C*) Fetal flat face by three-dimensional ultrasound. (*Lower, C–E*) Fetal MR images at the same gestation. Cobblestone lissencephaly with hypoplastic cerebellum, shallow sylvian fissures and agenesis of the corpus callosum is clearly demonstrated.

lissencephaly of the third trimester, similar to the 10- to 12-week brain, is shown in **Fig. 10**. The appearance of cobblestone lissencephaly with agenesis of the corpus callosum and hypoplastic cerebellum in late pregnancy is shown in **Fig. 11**. For specifying the type of disease, genetic mutational analysis is required to correlate between the abnormal sonographic/MR imaging finding and possible genetic cause. Significant overlap between the various phenotypic expressions of the above-listed categories exists and well-defined phenotype–genotype correlation is presently unavailable.

SCHIZENCEPHALY

This rare abnormality is characterized by congenital clefts in the cerebral mantle, lined by pia-ependyma, with communication between the subarachnoid space laterally and the ventricular system medially. Sixty three percent of cases are unilateral and 37% bilateral. The frontal region is affected in 44% of cases and the frontoparietal region in 30% of cases.[9,10] Few reports of prenatal sonographic diagnosis of schizencephaly are available.[11] **Fig. 12** demonstrates typical bilateral schizencephaly with the MR image clearly depicting gray matter lining the lesion.

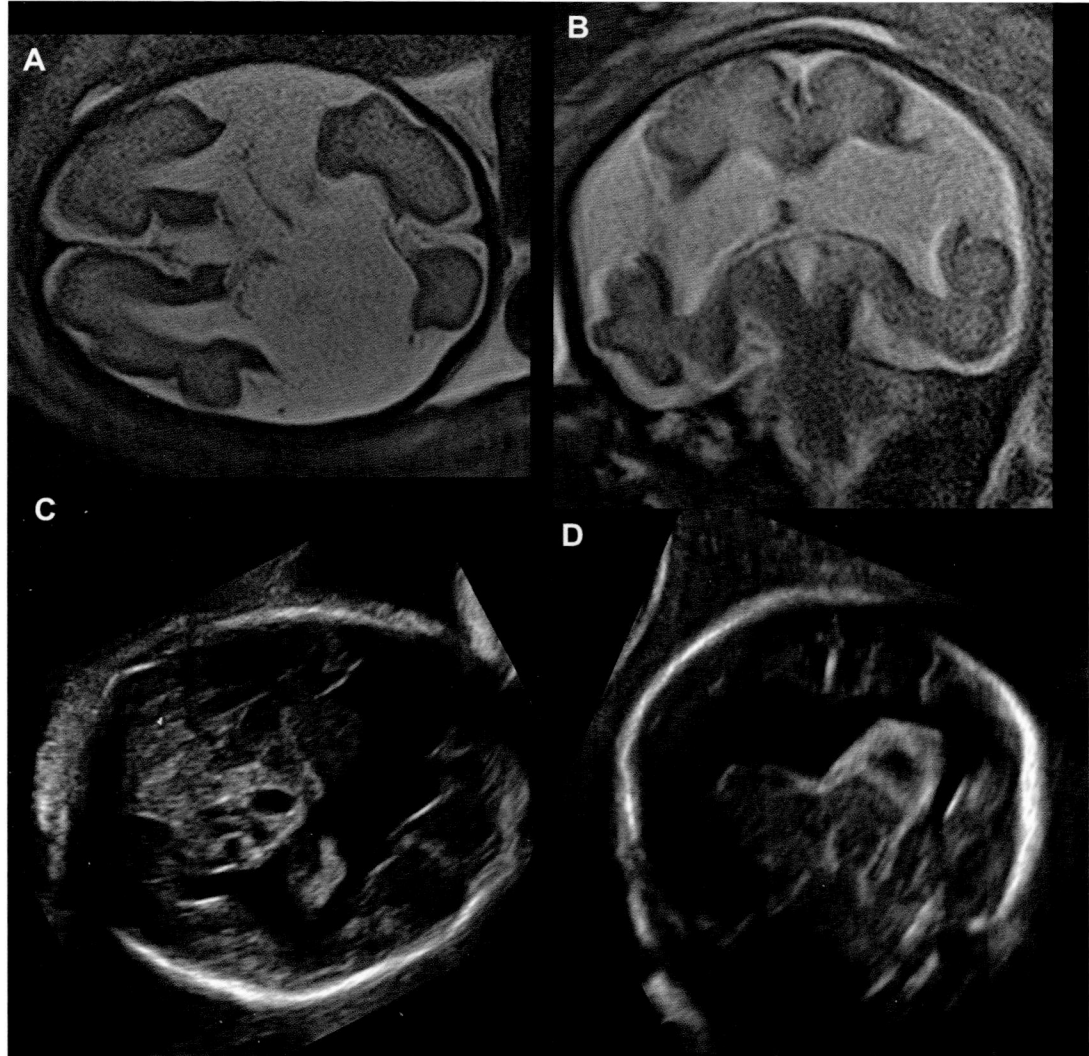

Fig. 12. Bilateral schizencephaly at 33 weeks of gestation. (*Upper left*, *A*) MR axial image. Bilateral schizencephaly, lined by pia-ependyma, is clearly demonstrated. (*Upper right*, *B*) MR coronal image. (*Lower left*, *C*) Sonographic axial and (*lower right*, *D*) coronal images.

SUMMARY

Prenatal diagnosis of migration disorder is among the most difficult challenges of an antenatal sonographic examination. Anterior coronal demonstration of the sylvian fissures is recommended as the screening of cortical development and maldevelopment. Once suspicion of a migration disorder develops, MR imaging is the preferred modality for demonstration of cortical development. Considering that migration disorders occur before fetal viability but detection of brain lesions is most commonly performed in the third trimester, this presents a diagnostic dilemma. Early detection of migration disorder with severe prognosis is among the central missions of fetal neuroimaging.

REFERENCES

1. Ross ME, Walsh CA. Human brain malformations and their lessons for neuronal migration. Annu Rev Neurosci 2001;24:1041–70.
2. Volpe JJ. Neuronal proliferation, migration, organization and myelination. Neurology of the newborn. 4th edition. USA: W.B. Saunders; 2001. p. 45–99.
3. Nadarajah B, Brunstrom JE, Grutzendler J, et al. Two modes of radial migration in early development of the cerebral cortex. Nat Neurosci 2001;4:143–50.
4. Righini A, Zirpoli S, Mrakic F, et al. Early prenatal MR imaging diagnosis of polymicrogyria. AJNR Am J Neuroradiol 2004;25:343–6.
5. Dobyns WB, Leventer RJ. Lissencephaly: the clinical and molecular genetic basis of diffuse malformations of neuronal migration. International Review of Child Neurology Series. In: Barth PG, editor. Disorder of neuronal migration. London: Mac Keith Press; 2003. p. 24–57.
6. McGahan JP, Grix A, Gerscovich EO. Prenatal diagnosis of lissencephaly: Miller-Dieker syndrome. J Clin Ultrasound 1994;22:560–3.
7. Greco P, Resta M, Vimercati A, et al. Antenatal diagnosis of isolated lissencephaly by ultrasound and magnetic resonance imaging. Ultrasound Obstet Gynecol 1998;12:276–9.
8. Kojima K, Suzuki Y, Seki K, et al. Prenatal diagnosis of lissencephaly (type II) by ultrasound and fast magnetic resonance imaging. Fetal Diagn Ther 2002;17:34–6.
9. Barkovich AJ, Kjos BO. Schizencephaly: correlation of clinical findings with MR characteristics. AJNR Am J Neuroradiol 1992;13:85–94.
10. Packard AM, Miller VS, Delgado MR. Schizencephaly: correlations of clinical and radiologic features. Neurology 1997;48:1427–34.
11. Denis D, Maugey-Laulom B, Carles D, et al. Prenatal diagnosis of schizencephaly by fetal magnetic resonance imaging. Fetal Diagn Ther 2001;16:354–9.

The Differential Diagnosis of Fetal Intracranial Cystic Lesions

Gustavo Malinger, MD[a,b,*], Edgardo Corral Sereño, MD[c], Tally Lerman-Sagie, MD[b,d]

KEYWORDS
- Intracranial cysts • Prenatal diagnosis • Ultrasound

Intracranial cystic lesions are frequently diagnosed by fetal ultrasound scan. They may come from many sources and involve different brain compartments. Although the most prevalent cysts are benign (choroid plexus cyst and arachnoid cyst) and do not affect development, the mere suspicion of a brain lesion during fetal life raises serious concerns in the prospective parents regarding the neurodevelopmental outcome of their child. It is therefore important to diagnose these lesions precisely and accordingly offer accurate counseling. The diagnosis and particularly the differential diagnosis and prognosis of intracranial cystic lesions identified in utero have not been studied as extensively as other more frequent brain anomalies (ie, ventriculomegaly), because of late development in some cases and presence in places that are not part of the routine ultrasound examination of the brain, such as the Sylvian fissure or ambiens cistern.

The purpose of this review is to present the differential diagnosis of intracranial cystic lesions in the context of prenatal counseling and prognostication.

Intracranial cysts may be classified into three different categories according to their place of origin: extra-axial, intraparenchymal, or intraventricular (**Table 1**).

CYSTS OF EXTRA-AXIAL ORIGIN

Arachnoid cysts are the most common type of cysts found on the brain surface. Usually the surface of these cysts is in contact with the dura and the external wall of the arachnoid. Arachnoid cysts are filled with cerebrospinal fluid, but they are usually not connected to the subarachnoid space. The walls of the cyst contain a thick layer of collagen and hyperplastic arachnoid cells but lack the trabecular processes characteristic of the normal arachnoid.[1] They may be found anywhere over the brain surface and also inside the ventricular system.

In children, common locations are the temporal fossa, the Sylvian fissure, and suprasellar or infratentorial regions. Interhemispheric cysts generally are associated with agenesis of the corpus callosum.

The prenatal diagnosis of arachnoid cysts has been reported on several occasions, including two large series.[2,3] Pierre-Khan and Sonigo[3] published their experience with 54 patients with arachnoid cysts; in 63% of their patients, the cysts were supratentorial, mostly placed in the interhemispheric fissure (25%), other common sites were the infratentorial region (22.2%) and the base of the cranium and the incisure. All the cysts were diagnosed after 20 weeks of gestation: 55%

---

[a] Prenatal Diagnosis Unit, Department of Obstetrics and Gynecology, Edith Wolfson Medical Center, Holon, Israel
[b] Sackler School of Medicine, Tel-Aviv University, Tel-Aviv, Israel
[c] Unidad de Ultrasonografia y Medicina Fetal, Servicio de Obsteticia y Ginecologia, Hospital Regional, Rancagua, Chile
[d] Pediatric Neurology Unit, Edith Wolfson Medical Center, Holon, Israel
* Corresponding author. Prenatal Diagnosis Unit, Department of Obstetrics and Gynecology, Edith Wolfson Medical Center, Holon, Israel.
E-mail address: gmalinger@gmail.com (G. Malinger).

Table 1
Differential diagnosis of fetal intracranial cystic lesions
Extra-axial cysts
Arachnoid cyst
Dural separation
Glioependymal cyst
Endodermal cyst
Cystic teratoma
Intraparenchymal cysts
Periventricular pseudocyst
Cystic periventricular leukomalacia
Porencephalic cyst
Brain cystic tumor
Intraventricular cysts
Choroid plexus cyst
Choroid plexus hemorrhage

between 20 and 30 weeks of gestation and the remaining 45% only after 30 weeks. In all their cases the initial suspicion was made by ultrasound, but they preferred magnetic resonance (MR) imaging to better delineate the structure and its surroundings and also to differentiate between malformative and acquired cysts. The authors stated that in the majority of the cases MR imaging did not modify the original diagnosis.

Diagnosis before 20 weeks of gestation has only been reported in infratentorial locations (**Fig. 1**).[4,5] Hogge and coworkers reported the prenatal diagnosis of an infratentorial arachnoid cyst in an 18-week fetus associated with an unbalanced X;9 translocation.[4] Bertelle and coworkers reported the presence of an isolated infratentorial cyst in a 13-week fetus with pathologic confirmation after termination of pregnancy at 15 weeks.[5]

Both the above-mentioned prenatal studies as well as postnatal studies found that the prognosis of these patients is generally good, even in those with hydrocephalus and requiring surgical drainage.[6,7] Although most arachnoid cysts are isolated findings (including secondary development of hydrocephalus) (**Fig. 2**), they may sometimes be associated with malformations of cortical development[8] (**Fig. 3**); metabolic diseases (glutaric aciduria type 1) or congenital hypothyroidism (personal experience). The prognosis will be according to the associated abnormalities. Therefore, in cases of prenatally diagnosed arachnoid cysts, it is important to follow-up longitudinally throughout the pregnancy, search for other brain anomalies considering MR imaging and check for glutaric aciduria type1 when the arachnoid cyst is in the opercular area.

The differential diagnosis includes neuroectodermal cysts, also known as glioependymal cysts,[9,10] endodermal cysts,[11] and even cystic teratoma.[12] All these diagnoses are extremely rare, and the working diagnosis in most cases of a cystic finding involving the brain meninges should be an arachnoid cyst. Even with the use of MR imaging, a correct diagnosis may be difficult to obtain as recently shown in a case report by Mühler and coworkers.[13] The authors suspected the presence of a porencephalic cyst in a fetus with unilateral ventriculomegaly, microcephaly, and a midline

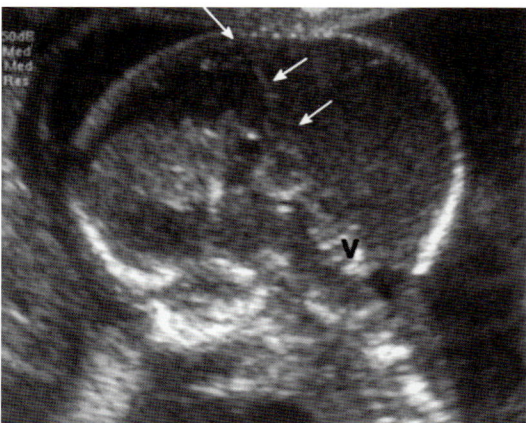

Fig. 1. Transvaginal midsagittal plane of the brain in a 15-week fetus shows a large infratentorial arachnoid cyst causing anterior displacement of the brain and the vermis. The *white arrows* show the position of the cystic wall; V, vermis.

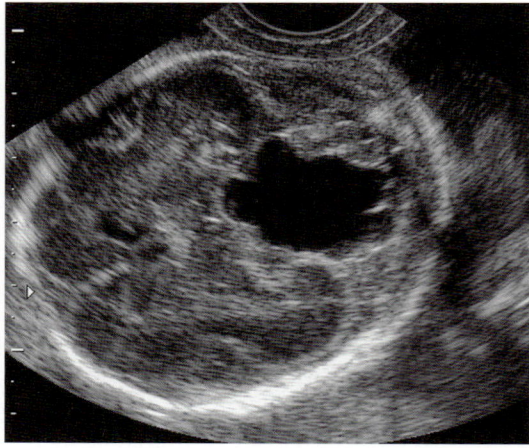

Fig. 2. Transvaginal axial plane of the brain in a 22-week fetus shows a prepontine arachnoid cyst. The size of the cyst remained stable throughout pregnancy, and the child was asymptomatic after birth.

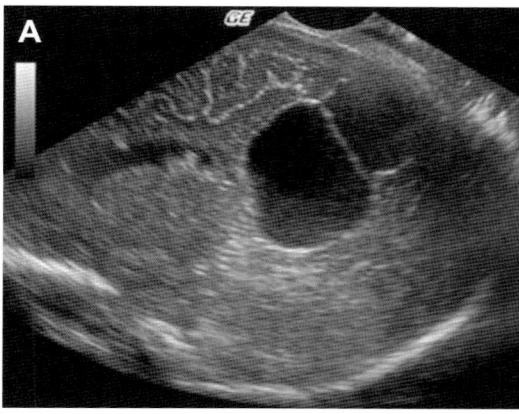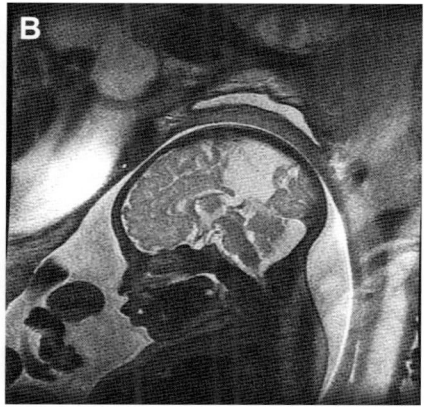

Fig. 3. Fetus at 40 weeks with periventricular heterotopia, pachygyria, and arachnoid cyst. (A) Transvaginal ultrasound scan shows the interhemispheric bilobate cyst. (B) MR imaging in a similar plane.

interhemispheric cyst, but the pathologic examination proved that the cyst was actually a glioependymal cyst.

INTRAPARENCHYMAL CYSTS

Cystic brain lesions may be the result of different types of insults (see **Table 1**). Cysts may develop as a consequence of hemorrhagic, ischemic, infectious, or tumoral processes. The prognosis depends on the presence of associated findings and on the extent and place of the insult.

Periventricular pseudocysts (PVPCs) usually are found at the level of the caudo-thalamic groove or close to the caudate nuclei; they may be unilateral or bilateral and unilocular or multilocular (**Fig. 4**).[14] These cysts probably develop after a small hemorrhagic event in the germinal matrix that upon resolution liquefies. PVPCs may be found in 1% of newborns, their diagnosis should prompt an investigation to rule out cytomegalovirus infection. Other less common etiologies found in association with PVPCs include cardiac malformations, chromosomal microdeletions (4p-), and metabolic or mitochondrial disorders. At least 50% of the cases represent isolated germinolytic events without development of any handicap in the affected children.

Prenatal diagnosis of PVPCs is possible based on the demonstration of the cysts adjacent to the lateral ventricle.[15] Although transabdominal axial planes generally are sufficient to raise the suspicion of the presence of PVPCs, transvaginal coronal and sagittal planes are more informative and help particularly in the differential diagnosis between this condition and periventricular leukomalacia.[15] In cases of associated growth retardation, fluorescent in situ hybridization for 4p- deletions is indicated; other tests should include maternal and, if necessary, amniotic fluid cytomegalovirus (CMV) status. Unfortunately, the prenatal diagnosis of most of the metabolic and mitochondrial disorders in which PVPCs may be present is not possible, and the suspicion of these diseases relies on familial history or the presence of associated anomalies.

Cystic periventricular leukomalacia (PVL) is most common in premature newborns, but it may occur also in full-term newborns after hypoxic–ischemic events.[16] Cystic PVL is the result of focal necrosis of the periventricular white matter, when the area of focal necrosis is large; the end result of the clastic process is cyst formation. The association between PVL and antenatal infection and inflammation has been studied extensively during the last decade;[17,18] maternal infection during pregnancy has been found to be very common among children developing cerebral palsy;[17] furthermore, histologic chorioamnionitis

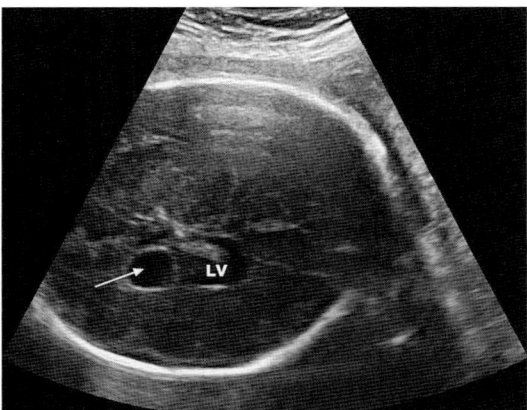

Fig. 4. Periventricular pseudocyst at 33 weeks of gestation (*white arrow*). Note the presence of mild ventriculomegaly. LV, lateral ventricle.

and congenital infection-related morbidity are more common among neonates with PVL than among those without PVL.[18]

Cystic lesions resembling PVL have been described in fetuses by the use of ultrasound scan and MR imaging,[19,20] but the differential diagnosis with PVPCs may be difficult as seen in two patients with pyruvate carboxylase deficiency in whom the investigators considered the cysts to be cystic PVL, whereas the actual diagnosis was PVPCs.[21] It is important to remember that PVL cysts are characteristically found on top of the lateral ventricles and not on their sides (**Fig. 5**).[15]

The authors have observed periventricular cysts in fetuses with metabolic, infective (mainly CMV)[22] and vascular conditions. The prognosis in these cases is usually reserved but some exceptions may occur.

Porencephalic cystic lesions occur after focal necrosis as a result of an ischemic event involving the vascular distribution of a single major cerebral vessel.[16]

Pilu and coworkers described the prenatal diagnosis of severe porencephaly in 10 fetuses diagnosed during the second half of pregnancy; in nine fetuses the cysts were connected with the lateral ventricles.[2] Termination of pregnancy was performed in three fetuses, perinatal death occurred in another three, and the remaining four children were delivered and suffer from severe neurodevelopmental delay.[2] Our group has recently reported the natural history of a probable focal arterial stroke diagnosed at 23 weeks evolving into a porencephalic cyst that eventually communicated with the lateral ventricle. After birth the child was found to have a familial leukoencephalopathy.[23] In another case, a large porencephalic cyst was found in association with brain disruption after a life-threatening car accident (**Fig. 6**).

Brain cystic tumors without the presence of solid components are extremely rare. A possible example of this type of tumor is the intraparenchymal choroid plexus papilloma (**Fig. 7**).

INTRAVENTRICULAR CYSTS

The most common type of intraventricular cysts is choroid plexus cysts (CPC). The choroid plexus is composed of secory neuroepithelium and is responsible for the production of cerebrospinal fluid (CSF). The choroid plexus epithelium is present all through the ventricular system but is more prominent in the lateral ventricles and usually is easily recognized by the use of ultrasound scan as a hyperechogenic structure starting from 8 weeks of gestation.[24]

Choroid plexus cysts are relatively common, and their prevalence ranges from 1% to 3.6% of pregnancies.[25] CPCs are sonolucent findings most commonly found in the body of the lateral ventricle choroid plexus (see **Fig. 1**), but have been described in other parts of the lateral ventricles and also in the third ventricle. Characteristically, they are not observed before 17 weeks, and in the majority of patients they disappear before 26 weeks of gestation. They may be unilateral or bilateral, nonseptated or septated. CPCs are not lined by epithelium but consist of a distended mesenchymal stroma with distended angiomatous interconnecting thin-walled capillaries.[26]

According to the current literature, CPCs are considered benign findings, and when isolated they do not increase the risk for chromosomal abnormalities. The observation of such a cyst should prompt the physician to perform a complete

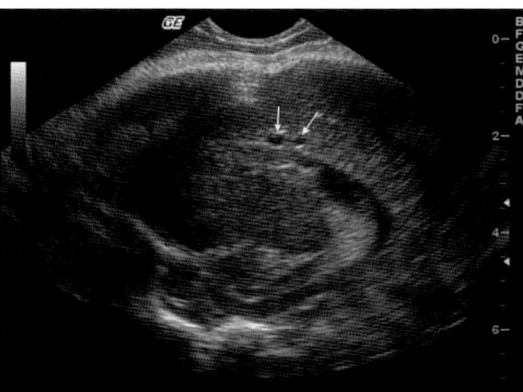

Fig. 5. Periventricular leukomalacia in a fetus referred at 28 weeks of gestation because of mild ventriculomegaly. Midsagittal plane shows the presence of two cysts on top of the lateral ventricles (*white arrows*).

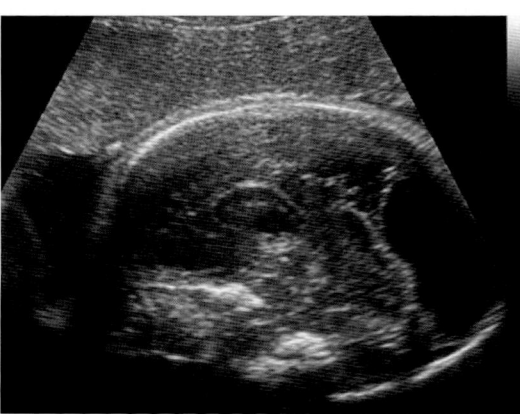

Fig. 6. Large porencephalic cyst at 31 weeks of gestation as a result of a car accident at 16 weeks.

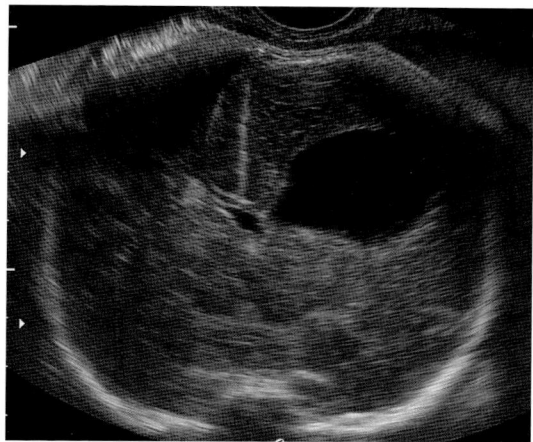

Fig. 7. Intraparenchymal cystic choroid plexus papilloma diagnosed at 35 weeks with normal development at the age of 20 months after surgery.

search for associated anomalies with particular attention to the heart, brain, and hands, because in cases caused by trisomy 18 there are malformations in these organs.[27] A possible association between CPC and trisomy 21 has been ruled out by almost all the well-designed published studies.[28]

Follow-up until their disappearance may be indicated because of the very rare possibility of the development of obstructive hydrocephaly caused by occlusion of CSF drainage through the Foramina of Monro in case of a large cyst.[29] The differential diagnosis should include the possibility of an intraventricular hemorrhage penetrating into the choroid plexus and other rare types of cysts that are seldom diagnosed in utero like colloid or ependymal cysts.

SUMMARY

Fetal intracranial cysts can be diagnosed during pregnancy by the use of ultrasound scan. The cysts can be found in different brain compartments and may be of diverse origins. Choroid plexus and arachnoid cysts are the most commonly diagnosed lesions and when isolated carry a good prognosis. Intraparenchymal cysts may have different etiologies, and the prognosis depends largely on the location and the extent of the lesion.

To give accurate counseling, it is fundamental to perform a detailed ultrasonographic examination, including multiplanar ultrasound scan of the brain, to search for additional anomalies. Fetal brain MR imaging may be complementary in difficult cases.

REFERENCES

1. Rengachary SS, Watanabe IJ. Ultrastructure and pathogenesis of intracranial arachnoid cysts. Neuropathol Exp Neurol 1981;40(1):61–83.
2. Pilu G, Falco P, Perolo A, et al. Differential diagnosis and outcome of fetal intracranial hypoechoic lesions: report of 21 cases. Ultrasound Obstet Gynecol 1997;9(4):229–36.
3. Pierre-Kahn A, Sonigo P. Malformative intracranial cysts: diagnosis and outcome. Childs Nerv Syst 2003;19(7–8):477–83.
4. Hogge WA, Schnatterly P, Ferguson JE II. Early prenatal diagnosis of an infratentorial arachnoid cyst: association with an unbalanced translocation. Prenat Diagn 1995;15(4):186–8.
5. Bretelle F, Senat MV, Bernard JP, et al. First trimester diagnosis of fetal arachnoid cyst: prenatal implication. Ultrasound Obstet Gynecol 2002; 20(4):400–2.
6. Zada G, Krieger MD, Mcnatt SA, et al. Pathogenesis and treatment of intracranial arachnoid cysts in pediatric patients younger than 2 years of age. Neurosurg Focus 2007;22(2):E1.
7. Pradilla G, Jallo G. Arachnoid cysts: case series and review of the literature. Neurosurg Focus 2007; 22(2):E7.
8. Malinger G, Kidron D, Schreiber L, et al. Prenatal diagnosis of malformations of cortical development by dedicated neurosonography. Ultrasound Obstet Gynecol 2007;29(2):178–91.
9. Hirano A, Hirano M. Benign cysts in the central nervous system: neuropathological observations of the cyst walls. Neuropathology 2004;24:1–7.
10. Pelkey TJ, Ferguson JE II, Veille JC, et al. Giant glioependymal cyst resembling holoprosencephaly on prenatal ultrasound: case report and review of the literature. Ultrasound Obstet Gynecol 1997; 9(3):200–3.
11. Chen PY, Wu CT, Lui TN, et al. Endodermal cyst presenting as a prenatally diagnosed large intracranial cyst. Case report and review of the literature. J Neurosurg 2007;106(6 Suppl):506–8.
12. Cassart M, Bosson N, Garel C, et al. Fetal intracranial tumors: a review of 27 cases. Eur Radiol 2008;[Epub ahead of print].
13. Mühler MR, Hartmann C, Werner W, et al. Fetal MRI demonstrates glioependymal cyst in a case of sonographic unilateral ventriculomegaly. Pediatr Radiol 2007;37(4):391–7.
14. Govaert P, de Vries LS. An atlas of neonatal brain sonography vol. 141–2. London: Mac Keith Press; 1997.
15. Malinger G, Lev D, Ben Sira L, et al. Congenital periventricular pseudocysts: prenatal sonographic appearance and clinical implications. Ultrasound Obstet Gynecol 2002;20(5):447–51.

16. Volpe JJ. Hypoxic-Ischemic encephalopathy: neuropathology and pathogenesis. In: Volpe JJ, editor. Neurology of the newborn. 5th edition. Philadelphia: Saunders; 2008. p. 347–99.
17. Bax M, Tydeman C, Flodmark O. Clinical and MRI correlates of cerebral palsy: the European Cerebral Palsy Study. JAMA 2006;296(13):1602–8.
18. Yoon BH, Park CW, Chaiworapongsa T. Intrauterine infection and the development of cerebral palsy. BJOG 2003;110(Suppl 20):124–7.
19. Garel C. Abnormalities of the fetal cerebral parenchyma: ischemic and hemorrhagic lesions. In: Garel C, editor. MRI of the fetal brain. Normal development and cerebral pathologies. Berlin: Springer; 2004. p. 247–62.
20. Ghi T, Brondelli L, Simonazzi G, et al. Sonographic demonstration of brain injury in fetuses with severe red blood cell alloimmunization undergoing intrauterine transfusions. Ultrasound Obstet Gynecol 2004; 23(5):428–31.
21. Brun N, Robitaille Y, Grignon A, et al. Pyruvate carboxylase deficiency: prenatal onset of ischemia-like brain lesions in two sibs with the acute neonatal form. Am J Med Genet 1999;84(2):94–101.
22. Malinger G, Lev D, Zahalka N, et al. Fetal cytomegalovirus infection of the brain: the spectrum of sonographic findings. AJNR Am J Neuroradiol 2003; 24(1):28–32.
23. Blumkin L, Watemberg N, Lev D, et al. Nonprogressive familial leukoencephalopathy with porencephalic cyst and focal seizures. J Child Neurol 2006;21(2):145–8.
24. Kennedy KA, Carey JC. Choroid plexus cysts: significance and current management practices. Semin Ultrasound CT MR 1993;4(1): 23–30.
25. Chinn DH, Miller EI, Worthy LM, et al. Sonographically detected fetal choroid plexus cysts. Frequency and association with aneuploidy. J Ultrasound Med 1991;10(5):255–8.
26. Kraus I, Jirásek JE. Some observations of the structure of the choroid plexus and its cysts. Prenat Diagn 2002;22(13):1223–8.
27. Snijders RJ, Shawa L, Nicolaides KH. Fetal choroid plexus cysts and trisomy 18: assessment of risk based on ultrasound findings and maternal age. Prenat Diagn 1994;14(12):1119–27.
28. Bromley B, Lieberman R, Benacerraf BR. Choroid plexus cysts: not associated with Down syndrome. Ultrasound Obstet Gynecol 1996;8(4): 232–5.
29. Nahed BV, Darbar A, Doiron R, et al. Acute hydrocephalus secondary to obstruction of the foramen of monro and cerebral aqueduct caused by a choroid plexus cyst in the lateral ventricle. Case report. J Neurosurg 2007;107(3 Suppl):236–9.

Magnetic Resonance Imaging Following Suspicion for Fetal Brain Anomalies

Alice B. Smith, Lt. Col, USAF, MC[a,b,*], Orit A. Glenn, MD[c]

KEYWORDS

- Fetal MR imaging • CNS anomalies
- Fetal brain • Sulcation • Ventriculomegaly
- Cortical malformation

Fetal ultrasound is considered the standard of care in the evaluation of fetal anomalies; however, limitations exist, including decreased visibility of fetal structures because of maternal body habitus, position of the fetal head, ossification of the fetal skull, and, in some cases, oligohydramnios. On the identification of a fetal brain anomaly by ultrasound, further evaluation is necessary to better define the anomaly and to rule out other associated anomalies. In the developing fetus, many brain structures are forming at around the same time; thus, the detection of one anomaly necessitates the evaluation for others. Fetal MR imaging is a complement to ultrasound and has several advantages, including visualization of the entire brain (as opposed to ultrasound where the upside cerebral hemisphere is often shadowed because of reverberations from overlying structures). MR imaging is also capable of assessing the sulcation pattern and developing cortex, which is difficult to visualize on ultrasound.[1–6] In addition, when an anomaly is detected, fetal MR imaging may provide better definition of the lesion because of improved contrast resolution and identify other lesions not visible on ultrasound.

Fetal MR imaging has been demonstrated to accurately detect anomalies within the second and third trimesters, providing additional information for prenatal counseling and delivery planning. In a study by Levine and colleagues of the central nervous system (CNS) of 145 fetuses, additional findings were found on MR imaging in 32%. Another study by Simon and colleagues[7] of 73 fetuses found that in 46% of cases the finding on fetal MR imaging changed patient management from what it would have been based on the ultrasound findings alone. When CNS anomalies are identified by ultrasound, MR imaging may demonstrate additional findings that may alter patient management.[6,8,9] Several studies have identified anomalies by MR imaging that were not visualized on ultrasound, including anomalies of sulcation, periventricular nodular heterotopia, callosal agenesis, periventricular white matter injury, cerebellar dysplasia, germinal matrix, and intraventricular hemorrhage.[7,10–14]

The opinions and assertions contained herein are the private views of the authors and are not to be construed as official or as reflecting the view of the Departments of the Army, Navy, Air Force, or Defense.
[a] Department of Radiologic Pathology, Armed Forces Institute of Pathology, 6825 16th Street NW, Washington, DC, USA
[b] Department of Radiology and Radiological Sciences, Uniformed Services University of the Health Sciences, 4301 Jones Bridge Road, Bethesda, MD 20814, USA
[c] Department of Radiology, Diagnostic Neuroradiology, University of California, San Francisco, Box 0628, L358, 505 Parnassus Avenue, San Francisco, CA 94143-0628, USA
* Corresponding author. Department of Radiology and Radiological Sciences, Uniformed Services University of the Health Sciences, 4301 Jones Bridge Road, Bethesda, MD 20814.
E-mail address: alsmith@usuhs.mil (A.B. Smith).

FETAL MR IMAGING TECHNIQUE AND LIMITATIONS

The use of fetal MR imaging began in the early 1980s in Europe, at which time fetal sedation was used. Since that time, improvements in technique have resulted in our ability to image the fetal brain without maternal or fetal sedation and thus in its increasing clinical use in the United States. Currently, most fetal MR imaging is performed using ultrafast T2-weighted MR imaging techniques known as single-shot fast spin echo (SSFSE) or half-Fourier acquired single-shot turbo spin echo (HASTE). These rapid pulse sequences allow acquisition of a single image in less than 1 second, reducing the artifact from fetal motion. In addition, T1-weighted images are used to visualize fat and hemorrhage, and gradient echo T2 images are used to visualize hemorrhage. Diffusion-weighted MR imaging can also now be performed in fetal MR imaging and is helpful in cases of suspected parenchymal injury, such as stroke or periventricular white matter injury. Diffusion-weighted MR imaging is also sensitive to maturational changes in the microstructure of fetal brain tissue, a process that normally occurs with increasing gestational age.[15,16] Diffusion tensor MR imaging provides even more information concerning tissue microstructure and maturational processes, although further technical advances are required before it can be successfully applied to fetuses.[17–19] MR spectroscopy is being investigated for the assessment of brain maturation and alterations in brain metabolism,[20–22] although it is limited by long acquisition time (4.5 minutes) and currently is only performed in the third trimester when the head is larger and engaged in the maternal pelvis.[23] Functional MR imaging is also being used in research protocols, but is not used in routine practice.[24–26] Fetal MR imaging is usually performed around 22 weeks' gestation, to decrease the effect of fetal motion that occurs with younger fetuses and the brain is larger, and, therefore, more easily assessed than at a younger gestational age.

A study by Blaicher and colleagues[27] found that the diagnostic accuracy increases with gestational age, and concluded that fetal MR imaging should be performed from 20 weeks onward, although we have found 22 weeks to be the optimal age for performing fetal MR imaging.

Patients are imaged on a 1.5 Tesla scanner using an eight-channel torso phased array coil, which is placed over the mother's abdomen. Preferably, the patient is imaged in the supine position, allowing for optimal coil geometry. Ultrafast SSFSE images (TR 4000, TE 90, FOV 24 cm, matrix 192 × 160) are obtained in coronal, axial, and sagittal planes, and 3-mm slice thickness is used for the brain (2 mm for the spine). No sedation is given to the mother, but she is instructed not to eat for 4 hours before the examination, because this tends to decrease the frequency of fetal movement. In addition, the patient is screened for any contraindications to MR imaging before the examination.

In addition to fetal motion, limitations of fetal MR imaging include the small size of the structure being evaluated combined with increased distance of the structure from the receiver coil, which limits the resolution. Improvements in coil technology, such as parallel imaging with increased number of channels, are resulting in the reduction in these limitations. Maternal claustrophobia and discomfort from lying still for the study period are also problems, because the MR imaging examination typically lasts at least 45 minutes. If the mother cannot lie on her back, she can be imaged in the left lateral decubitus position, which may ease discomfort, although this does result in decreased image quality.

MR IMAGING SAFETY

MR imaging of the fetus is considered to be safe; however, studies on the safety of MR imaging in pregnant women are limited. Follow-up studies of children who underwent fetal MR imaging have thus far demonstrated no long-term adverse effects; however, these studies have been limited by small sample size.[28–30] Because the effect of MR imaging on the developing fetus has not been determined, it is not recommended in the first trimester to avoid the potential risk for the magnetic fields interfering with organogenesis. Biologic effects, miscarriage, acoustic noise exposure, and heating effects are the potential risks from exposure to the magnetic field. Studies using pregnant animals and animal fetuses have not provided a consensus as to risk, and whether or not the information can be applied to humans is uncertain because the equipment and scanner parameters were variable in these studies.[31–35] To provide guidance for imaging, a 2002 American College of Radiology white paper states, "Pregnant patients can be accepted to undergo MR images at any stage of pregnancy if, in the determination of a Level Two MR Personnel –designated attending radiologist, the risk-benefit ratio to the patient warrants that the study be performed."[36] All pregnant women should undergo counseling and sign a consent form before MR imaging.

In addition, the use of gadolinium for fetal MR imaging has been avoided. Gadolinium is a "rare earth" element, which is toxic when it is in an unbound state. When bound to a chelating agent it is no longer toxic, as in the form used as an intravenous contrast agent (gadolinium-DTPA). Gadolinium crosses the placenta, is exced in the urine of the fetus, and can then be swallowed.[37] It thus remains within the fetal environment where there is the potential for it to become unbound, and there is concern that in the unbound form it may have a teratogenic effect. Gadolinium is labeled as a pregnancy category C by the Food and Drug Administration because of lack of epidemiologic studies evaluating exposure in the first trimester. A recent study reported by De Santis and colleagues[38] in 2007 of 26 women who received gadolinium during the first trimester found no adverse pregnancy or neonatal outcome. The current recommendation for using gadolinium during pregnancy is only when the potential benefit to the mother outweighs the potential risk to the fetus. There are few, if any, situations in which gadolinium would provide additional useful information in the evaluation of fetal brain anomalies and its benefit would outweigh its risk.

ABNORMALITIES OF THE FETAL BRAIN

An understanding of the normal development of the fetal brain on MR imaging is essential for the identification of anomalies and several excellent reviews are available.[39–46] In brief, the formation of sulci occurs in an organized and time-specific manner, with primary sulcation complete by about 32 to 34 weeks. The appearance of the sulci on fetal MR imaging lags behind that seen in fetal autopsy by a mean of 1.9 ± 2.2 weeks, which most likely reflects the limitations of MR resolution.[40,41] In addition, the depth and complexity of a sulcus progresses with increasing gestational age, and thus it is important to evaluate the appearance and the morphology of the sulci on fetal MR imaging (**Fig. 1**; **Table 1**).

In addition to evaluating the sulcation pattern, fetal MR imaging also allows evaluation of the brain parenchyma. Normally, a multilayered pattern is present in the developing parenchyma from about 20 to 28 gestational weeks, which represents different developing layers in the fetal brain (**Fig. 2**). The multilayered pattern disappears in a topographically and timely organized manner that corresponds to known histologic changes in developing brain layers with increasing gestational age. It disappears from the depths of the sulci and then from the crests of the gyri and from different regions of the brain in time-specific fashion as the sulci form.[47,48] Prominent subarachnoid spaces are also normally noted in the fetus, especially before 30 weeks, in comparison with the term infant. A complete discussion of the maturational changes of the fetal brain is beyond the scope of this article, but it is important to stress that knowledge of the gestational age of the fetus is critical to proper image interpation.

Developmental anomalies of the fetal brain have various causes, including chromosomal, infectious, and destructive. Fetal brain structures are developing at approximately the same time; therefore, the presence of one anomaly should prompt the search for others. Primary indications for MR imaging of the fetal brain are for the evaluation of ventriculomegaly and other CNS anomalies visualized on prenatal ultrasound, and to assess the fetal brain when there is a risk for fetal brain damage, such as in complicated monochorionic twin pregnancies.[49–51]

VENTRICULOMEGALY

Ventriculomegaly is defined as enlargement of the ventricular atrium greater than 10 mm at the level of the thalami in the axial plane with the measurement being made through the posterior aspect of the glomus.[52] The size of the ventricular atria remains relatively constant from 15 to 35 weeks; the brain, however, enlarges so the relative size of the ventricles compared with the brain decreases. Ventriculomegaly is the most frequently detected intracranial anomaly on prenatal ultrasound, and frequently results in referral for further evaluation by MR imaging, which may be able determine the cause or associated anomalies not detected on ultrasound.[53] A study by Levine and colleagues[54] of the similarity of ventricular size measured on ultrasound compared with MR imaging in the axial plane demonstrated minimal differences with the measurements being within 2 mm of each other. In a study by Garel and Alberti,[55] measurements of ventricular size in the coronal plane on ultrasound and MR imaging were similar.

There are numerous causes of ventriculomegaly, and prognosis is related, at least in part, to the presence of other anomalies. The cause may be obstruction, destructive processes, or developmental or chromosomal abnormalities. In mild ventriculomegaly (atrial size 10–15 mm), reported associated anomalies, both neuronal and somatic, may be present in up to 75% of cases.[53,56] These anomalies include neuronal heterotopia, lissencephaly, intraventricular hemorrhage, and neural tube defects. In a study by Bromley and colleagues[57] of patients who had borderline mild ventriculomegaly (10–12 mm), the frequency of associated anomalies decreased to 39%. Frequently, the ventriculomegaly is isolated (ie, no other additional extra- or intracerebral anomalies),

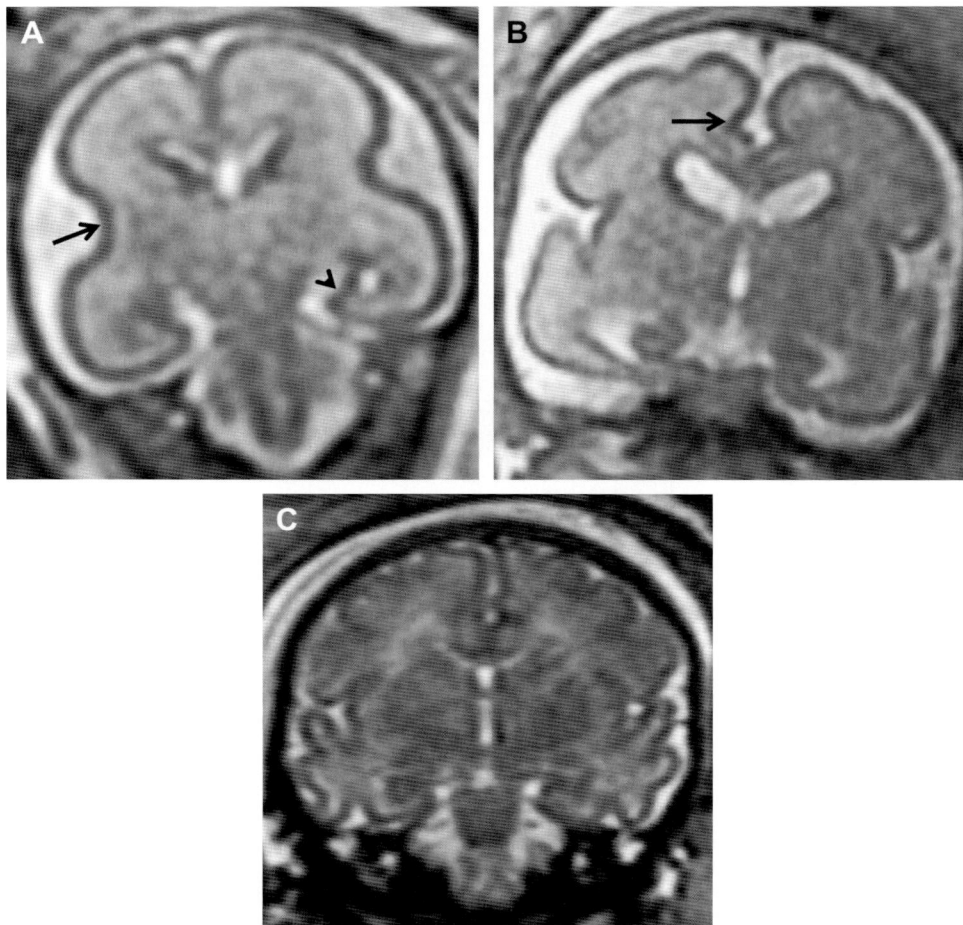

Fig. 1. Progression of normal sulcation. (*A*) Coronal T2 SSFSE of a 23-week estimated gestational age (EGA) fetus demonstrates formation of the sylvian fissure (*arrow*), and hippocampal sulcus (*arrowhead*). Note the prominence of the cerebrospinal fluid (CSF) space. (*B*) Coronal T2 SSFSE of a 29-week EGA fetus reveals further development of the sylvian fissure. In addition, the cingulate sulcus is identified (*arrow*) and further definition of the hippocampal sulcus. (*C*) Coronal T2 SSFSE of a 34-week EGA fetus shows the complete primary sulcation pattern. Note the decreased prominence of the CSF space.

and, to date, the impact on the fetus's postnatal neurodevelopmental outcome for mild, isolated cases is still not completely understood. Previous studies reported the incidence of developmental delay in cases of prenatal isolated mild ventriculomegaly (IMVM) to range from 0% to 36%.[56,58–61] In cases in which the atrial diameter is less than 12 mm, several studies have found a lower risk for developmental delay, especially if the fetus is male.[56,59,61,62] In a more recent study by Falip and colleagues[63] of postnatal clinical and imaging follow-up of 101 infants who had isolated mild ventriculomegaly on prenatal ultrasound and fetal MR imaging, 94% of infants who had ventricular size of 10 to 11.9 mm had favorable outcome, and 85% of those who had ventricular size of 12 to 15 mm had a favorable outcome, although the difference between the two groups was not statistically significant. No difference in prognosis was found between uni- and bilateral IMVM or between stable, progressive, and resolved IMVM, and prognosis was independent of the gestation age at diagnosis and gender. In addition, they reported white matter abnormalities detected only on postnatal MR imaging in two thirds of the infants who had poor outcome.[63]

Because the prognosis for fetuses who have ventriculomegaly is related to the presence of other anomalies, a search for associated anomalies is necessary. Studies have shown a false-negative rate for detection of associated anomalies with prenatal ultrasound in experienced prenatal

Table 1
Expected normal appearance of primary sulci for gestational age

Sulcus	Gestational Age (wk)
Parietoccipital sulcus	20–23
Calcarine sulcus	24–25
Callosal sulcus	22–23
Hippocampal sulcus	22–23
Cingulate sulcus	24–25
Central sulcus	27
Superior temporal sulcus	27
Precentral sulci	27
Postcentral sulci	28

Gestational age at which sulci are present in ≥75% of fetuses.
Data from Garel C, Chantrel E, Brisse H, et al. Fetal cerebral cortex: normal gestational landmarks identified using prenatal MR imaging. AJNR Am J Neuroradiol 2001;22(1):184–9.

diagnostic centers to be 10% to 25%.[56,64] Examples of sonographically occult lesions include developmental anomalies, such as agenesis of the corpus callosum, cerebellar dysplasia, and cortical dysplasia, and the sequelae of destructive processes, such as periventricular leukomalacia, and subependymal and intraventricular hemorrhage.[6,11,12,65] In addition, sonography has been noted to be limited in its ability to detect associated anomalies in the presence of ventriculomegaly.[61,66] Fetal MR imaging is capable of identifying additional anomalies in up to 50% of cases of fetal ventriculomegaly, thereby providing additional information for the parents.[6,8–10]

CALLOSAL AGENESIS

Fetal MR imaging provides an excellent means for evaluation of the corpus callosum because of its capability of imaging it in the sagittal and coronal planes. It has better specificity in evaluation of the corpus than ultrasound. One study demonstrated that an intact corpus was identified in 20% of fetuses who were suspected to have an abnormal corpus on ultrasound.[11] Ultrasound identifies agenesis by the characteristic parallel configuration of the lateral ventricles and colpocephaly,[67] and by the absence of a cavum septum pellucidum. Occasionally, on second and third trimester ultrasounds, the fornix mimics the cavum septum pellucidum resulting in a missed diagnosis of callosal agenesis.[68]

In addition to absence of the corpus callosum, other associated findings on fetal MR imaging include colpocephaly, abnormal configuration of the frontal horns of the lateral ventricles that have a "steer's horns" appearance on the coronal view, and, in older fetuses, a radial pattern of the medial sulci with extension to the third ventricle, which results from a persistent eversion of the cingulate gyrus (**Fig. 3**). The corpus callosum develops from the commissural plate, as do the anterior and hippocampal commissures; therefore, anomalies of the corpus callosum are

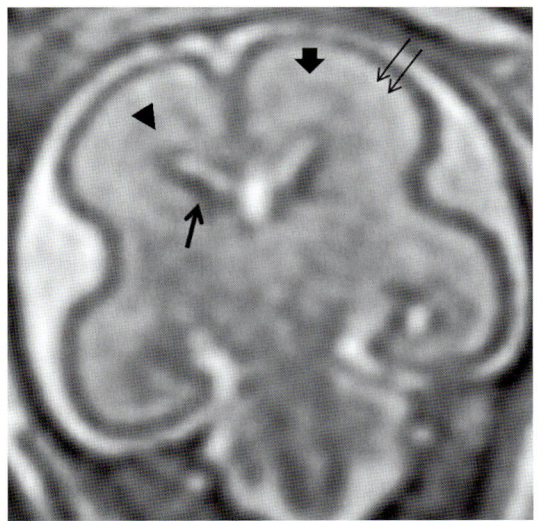

Fig. 2. Multilayer pattern. Coronal T2 SSFSE of a 23-week EGA fetus demonstrates the multilayer pattern. The germinal matrix (*thin arrow*) is the deepest layer. The periventricular zone (*arrowhead*) is adjacent to the germinal matrix. The more superficial layers are the subventricular and intermediate zones (*thick arrow*), and the subplate, which is recognized as a band of high signal (*double arrows*). The developing cortex and marginal zone are the most superficial layers.

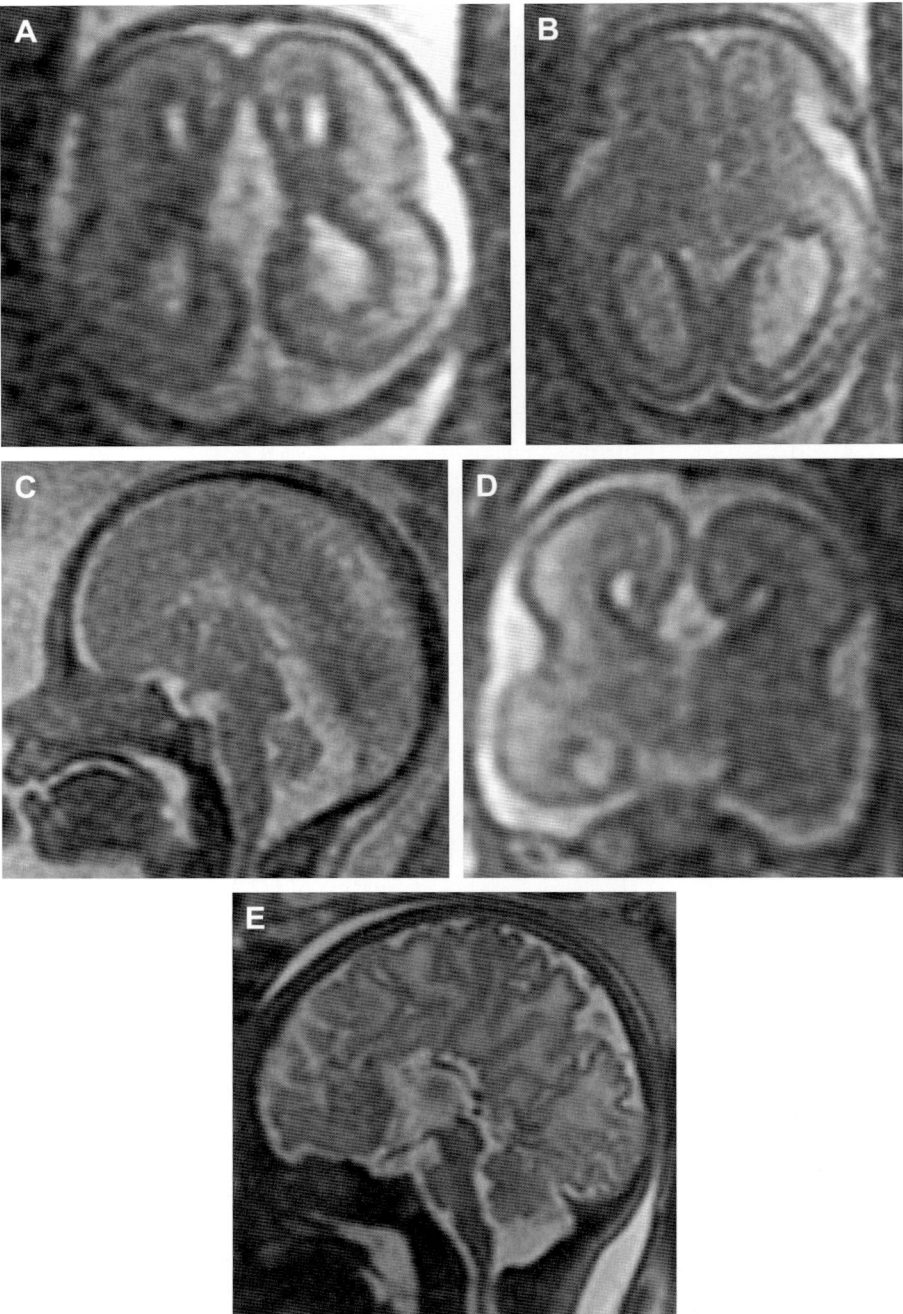

Fig. 3. Agenesis of the corpus callosum. (A) Axial T2 SSFSE of a 22-week EGA fetus demonstrates a parallel configuration of the lateral ventricles. (B) Axial T2 SSFSE of a 22-week EGA fetus reveals prominence of the occipital horns of the lateral ventricles consistent with colpocephaly. (C) Sagittal T2 SSFSE of a 34-week EGA fetus demonstrates absence of the corpus callosum. (D) Coronal T2 SSFSE of a 22-week EGA fetus reveals absence of the corpus callosum with the resultant abnormal configuration ("steer's horns") of the frontal horns. (E) Sagittal T2 SSFSE of a 34-week EGA fetus demonstrates absence of the corpus callosum. At this gestational age the radial pattern of the sulci extending to midline is appreciated.

frequently associated with anomalies of the anterior and hippocampal commissures. Typically, these are aplastic or hypoplastic, but occasionally they may be enlarged; enlargement of the hippocampal commissure may be mistaken for the splenium of the corpus callosum.[39] In addition, knowledge of the normal development of the corpus callosum helps differentiate a hypoplastic corpus callosum from one that is secondarily destroyed. In general, the corpus develops in a front-to-back pattern with the genu forming first, then the body, splenium, and, finally, the rostrum. A deviation from this pattern may indicate the presence of holoprosencephaly (dysplasia of the corpus callosum with only the posterior aspect formed), or cerebral lesions in regions sending fibers across the corpus callosum (porencephalies, schizencephaly). The presence of callosal/commissural anomalies is an important clinical finding. The belief that isolated callosal agenesis is of no clinical significance has been challenged. In a study by Moutard and colleagues[69] of children who had prenatally diagnosed isolated agenesis of the corpus callosum, behavioral and cognitive abnormalities became more apparent as the children reached school age. In the future, diffusion-tensor MR imaging may provide a means for further evaluation of callosal agenesis.

Agenesis of the corpus callosum is associated with other CNS anomalies and more than 70 different syndromes, and identification of associated anomalies is greater with fetal MR imaging than ultrasound.[14,70] In a study of children by Hetts and colleagues,[71] agenesis of the corpus callosum was frequently (>50%) associated with reduction in white matter volume and cortical malformations, the most frequent of which is heterotopia. Heterotopia was identified on postnatal imaging in 29% of these patients, and hypogenesis of the corpus callosum was associated with heterotopia in 21%. Autopsy studies have demonstrated additional CNS anomalies in up to 85% of patients who have callosal agenesis.[72] In addition to gray matter heterotopia, these include Chiari II malformation, schizencephaly, Dandy-Walker malformation, and encephaloceles.[73] Evaluation for these associated anomalies is critical, because their presence is associated with a higher incidence of neurodevelopmental disability, and if findings are present that suggest a genetic syndrome this provides important information for counseling the parents regarding future pregnancies.[14,73,74] Abnormalities of the hippocampi are also associated with callosal agenesis. Incomplete inversion of the hippocampal formation may be seen. The temporal horns may develop a keyhole shape as a result of deficiency of the hippocampal formation, which can be seen in older fetuses with callosal agenesis.

ABNORMALITIES OF CORTICAL DEVELOPMENT

Cortical malformations are important imaging findings that are frequently associated with neurodevelopmental abnormalities, and studies have demonstrated that fetal MR imaging has the ability to detect cortical malformations that are not detected on ultrasound.[6,13,14] Abnormalities of cortical development can be classified by the stage of development during which they occur as abnormal neuronal and glial proliferation or apoptosis (including focal transmantle cortical dysplasia with balloon cells, microlissencephaly, schizencephaly, and hemimegalencephaly), abnormal neuronal migration (lissencephaly, heterotopia, polymicrogyria, and congenital muscular dystrophy), or abnormal cortical organization (polymicrogyria and focal cortical dysplasia without balloon cells). Other causes of cortical malformations include exogenous (maternal alcohol or drug abuse) or endogenous (metabolic disorders) toxins, the sequelae of infection (cytomegalovirus) or ischemia (monochorionic twinning complications). Classification of anomalies can be problematic because of the likelihood of multiple anomalies. Identifying malformations of cortical development by MR imaging may be difficult in fetuses less than 25 weeks, because few sulci and gyri are normally seen at this stage.[1] When assessing cortical malformations it is beneficial to obtain follow-up MR imaging, because the appearance of cortical malformations changes with increased fetal age.

ABNORMAL NEURONAL AND GLIAL PROLIFERATION OR APOPTOSIS
Transmantle Cortical Dysplasia with Balloon Cells

In cases of focal transmantle cortical dysplasia with balloon cells there is a focal region of abnormal cortical lamination in which the normal six-layered appearance of the cerebral cortex is disturbed. The abnormality extends through the entire cerebral mantle, and on histologic examination abnormal cells, including balloon cells, atypical glia, and large dysplastic neurons, are seen within the cerebral cortex and underlying white matter.[6,75] On imaging, focal transmantle cortical dysplasia can be visualized as an area of low signal on T2 SSFE that is wedge-shaped and extends from the pial surface to the ventricular surface.

Tuberous sclerosis is an autosomal dominant phakomatosis (80% of cases are de novo mutations) in which there are transmantle dysplasias and cortical tubers that on imaging and pathology are identical to focal cortical dysplasia with balloon cells (**Fig. 4**).[39] Referral to a geneticist for a patient who has evidence of transmantle cortical dysplasia is indicated to rule out the possibility of tuberous sclerosis. A search for other manifestations of tuberous sclerosis, such as subependymal nodules, should be undertaken. MR imaging can also be used to evaluate the heart, because rhabdomyomas may be seen in at least 60% of patients who have tuberous sclerosis.[76,77]

Microlissencephaly

Fetuses who have microlissencephaly demonstrate a small head circumference (more than three standard deviations from normal) resulting from a reduction in proliferation of neurons and glia in the germinal zones.[39] These fetuses have too few gyri and shallow sulci, and the volume of white matter is reduced. When suspected, it is necessary to evaluate for genetic causes and potential acquired causes, such as infection, ischemia, inborn errors of metabolism, toxins, and radiation exposure.

Schizencephaly

Schizencephaly is a term to describe a gray matter–lined cleft extending from the brain surface to the ependymal lining that may result from a genetic anomaly (mutation of the EMX2 homeobox gene—although this has been disputed recently) or a transmantle injury occurring in the second trimester (**Fig. 5**).[39,78] When open lipped it is easily identified, but closed-lipped schizencephaly may be more difficult to visualize, although it is typically associated with dimpling of the ventricular surface at the site of the schizencephaly. When unilateral, assessment of the contralateral cortex is important, because there may be an associated mirror image cortical malformation. The septum pellucidum is almost always absent when the clefts are bilateral. The severity of the patient's symptoms depends on the amount of involved brain.

Hemimegalencephaly

Hemimegalencephaly is a hamartomatous overgrowth of all or part of a cerebral hemisphere, in which the affected portion has little or no function. Affected children typically have intractable epilepsy and severe developmental delay.[79] Hemimegalencephaly can be difficult to detect prenatally and slight brain asymmetry may not be detected by ultrasound.[43] Fetal MR imaging may be more sensitive to the detection of hemimegalencephaly because abnormal signal within the white matter and an overlying abnormal gyral pattern may be seen.[43]

ABNORMAL NEURONAL MIGRATION
Classical Lissencephaly

Lissencephaly is a paucity of gyral and sulcal development, resulting from the arrest of normal neuronal migration. Patients have either agyria (no gyration) or pachygyria (broad, simplified gyri).

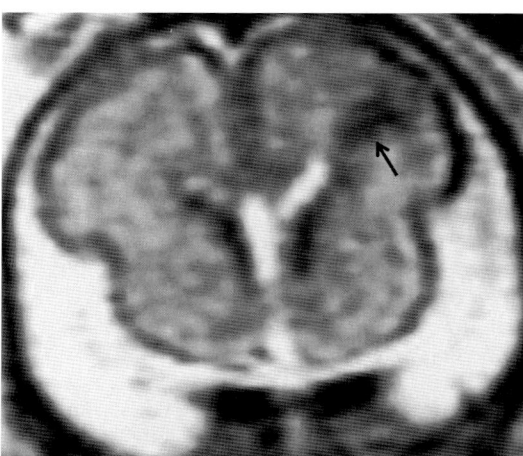

Fig. 4. Tuberous sclerosis. Coronal T2 SSFSE of a 26-week EGA fetus demonstrates a focal wedge-shaped area of low signal extending from the cortex to the lateral ventricle. Both focal cortical dysplasia with balloon cells and the subcortical tubers of tuberous sclerosis have this imaging appearance. In this case, the patient had tuberous sclerosis.

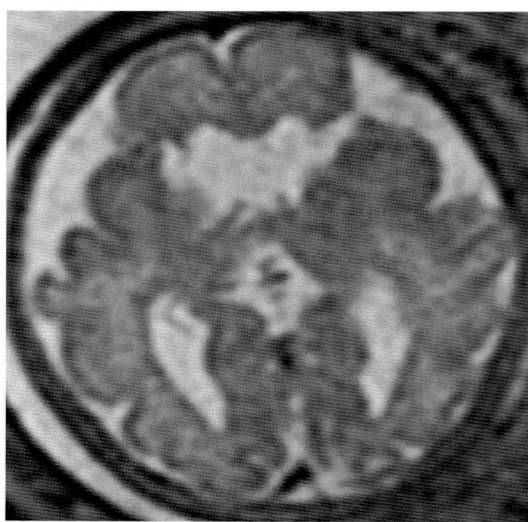

Fig. 5. Schizencephaly. Coronal T2 SSFSE of a 33-week EGA fetus reveals bilateral, symmetric clefts involving the frontal lobes consistent with open-lipped schizencephaly.

Agyria is seen in the Miller-Dieker syndrome, which is linked to chromosome 17 and involves the LISI gene. Posterior pachygyria is also associated with chromosome 17 deletions, and anterior pachygyria is seen in the X-linked form (associated with mutations of the doublecortin gene located on chromosome X). Fetal MR imaging is beneficial in patients who have a family history of lissencephaly. In the normal development of the fetus, the sulci are visualized at predictable times by MR imaging (see **Table 1**). Knowledge of the estimated gestational age is critical when assessing sulcal development. A delay in sulcation should raise the suspicion of lissencephaly and a follow-up fetal MR imaging may be indicated to confirm persistent sulcation delay. In classical lissencephaly, normal sulcation is not visualized and the sylvian fissures remain shallow (**Fig. 6**).[23] There is also a thickened deep cortical layer, representing a band of arrested neurons, which is separated from a thin outer cortical layer by a zone of white matter.[39,40] Histologically, a thick four-layer cortex is noted consisting of the cortical plate and a thick layer of heterotopic cells.[43]

Heterotopia

Gray matter heterotopia result from under-migration of neurons; they can be described as nodular or laminar and by their location (periventricular or subcortical). Subependymal heterotopia can be identified as focal or diffuse areas of low signal along the ventricular lining (**Fig. 7**). These protrude into the ventricles, and should not be confused

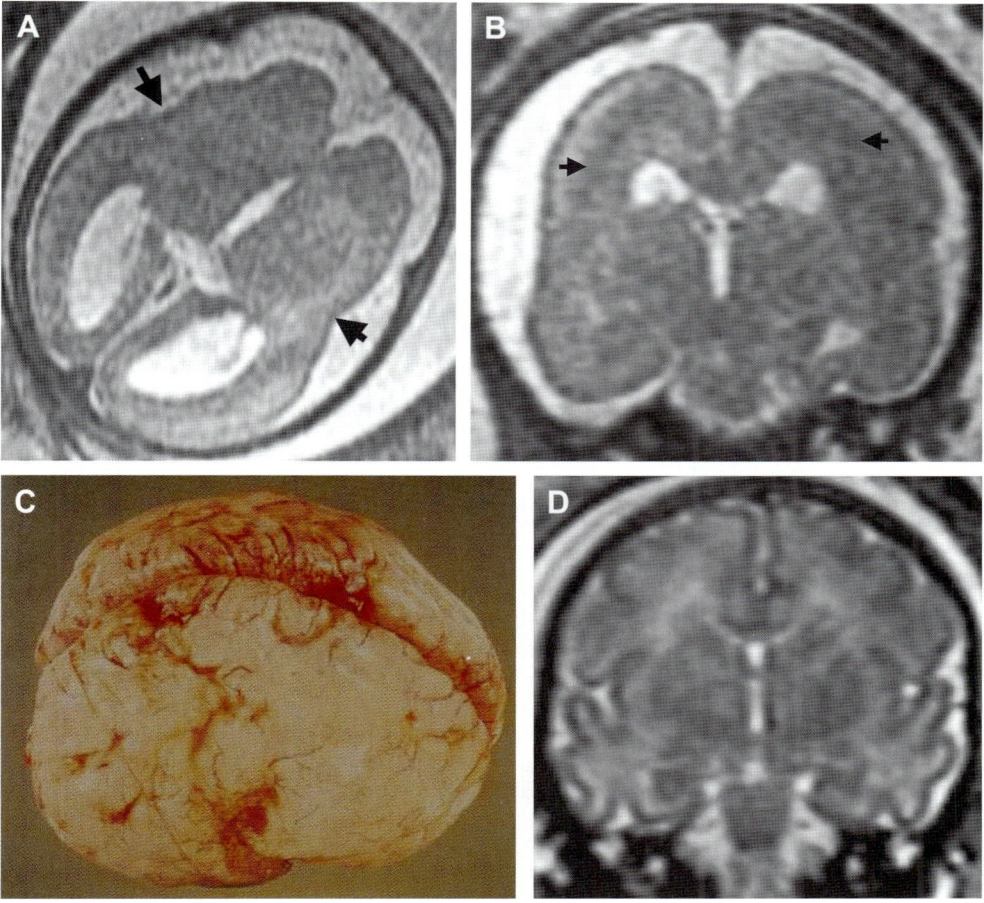

Fig. 6. Classical lissencephaly. (A) Axial T2 SSFSE of a 34-week EGA fetus demonstrates a shallow sylvian fissure (*arrows*) and paucity of the other primary fissures. Notice the prominence of the CSF spaces. (B) Coronal T2 SSFSE of the same fetus demonstrates shallow sylvian fissures and absence of the other primary sulci. An abnormal multilayer pattern with thick band of low signal in the developing white matter is seen (*arrows*). (C) Photograph of gross specimen of a brain with lissencephaly from an autopsy at 38 gestational weeks demonstrates the absence of normal sulcation. (D) Coronal T2 SSFSE of a 34-week EGA fetus reveals the normal sulcation pattern expected for this stage of gestation.

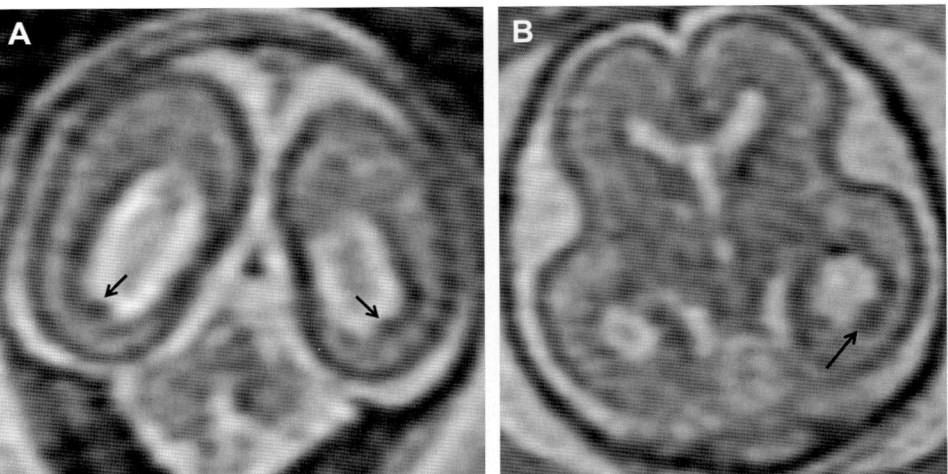

Fig. 7. Subependymal heterotopia. Coronal (A) and axial (B) T2 SSFSE of a 22-week EGA fetus demonstrates nodularity along the ventricular surface (arrows) consistent with subependymal heterotopia.

with germinal matrix, which is also low in signal but does not protrude into the ventricle. In addition, the germinal matrix begins to involute after 26 to 28 weeks. If the subependymal heterotopia is bilateral and diffuse, this is associated with an X-linked disorder that is lethal in males. Presence of heterotopia should be confirmed in two imaging planes. In addition, subependymal heterotopia are indistinguishable from the subependymal nodules seen in tuberous sclerosis; therefore a thorough search for other manifestations of tuberous sclerosis (cortical tubers, transmantle dysplasia, and cardiac rhabdomyoma) is necessary. Heterotopia, however, are much more common than tuberous sclerosis. Band heterotopia is frequently not imaged because of lack of ultrasound abnormalities.[43]

Polymicrogyria

Polymicrogyria results when neurons distribute abnormally in the cortex resulting in multiple small gyri. Suspicion of polymicrogyria should occur when sulci are present that are not expected according to gestational age, and if an irregular surface of the brain is noted.[43] Polymicrogyria is frequently perisylvian, and the appearance of a thickened cortex in this region may be a clue to its presence. In other regions an appearance of too many sulci in a less mature fetus or too few sulci or abnormally located sulci in a more mature fetus should be a clue to the presence of polymicrogyria (**Fig. 8**).[23,80] Two forms of polymicrogyria have been described based on microscopy and include a four-layered form and an unlayered form.[81] The layered form of polymicrogyria is believed to be attributable to postmigrational events, whereas the unlayered form is believed to be attributable to events that occur before the end of neuroblast migration (before 17 weeks).[81] Currently, imaging features cannot distinguish layered from unlayered polymcirogyria. Polymicrogyria is frequently associated with chromosomal anomalies. Other causes of polymicrogyria include the sequelae of infection (cytomegalovirus), ischemia (as can occur in monochorionic co-twin demise), exposure to exogenous toxins, and endogeneous toxins (inherent metabolic disorders).[39,43]

Congenital Muscular Dystrophy

Congenital muscular dystrophies are a heterogeneous group of disorders characterized by hypotonia, weakness, and, frequently, congenital contractures with an autosomal recessive mode of inheritance. Brain involvement in these disorders occurs in approximately 50%, and includes cobblestone (type II) lissencephaly that results from a disorder in neuronal migration in which the migrating neurons are not able to dissociate from the radial glial fibers that guide them to their final location, leading to an overmigration of neurons.[82] The most severe form, Walker-Warburg syndrome, demonstrates a cobblestone cortex and has a classic dorsal "kink" at the pontomesencephalic junction along with fusion of the superior and inferior colliculi, which can be identified by fetal MR imaging (**Fig. 9**). Prenatally, ventriculomegaly with cerebellar hypoplasia are the most common findings on ultrasound.[83] A variable degree of callosal hypogenesis is also present and can be detected prenatally. Fetal MR imaging can identify the lissencephaly and cerebellar and brainstem abnormalities. These patients also have

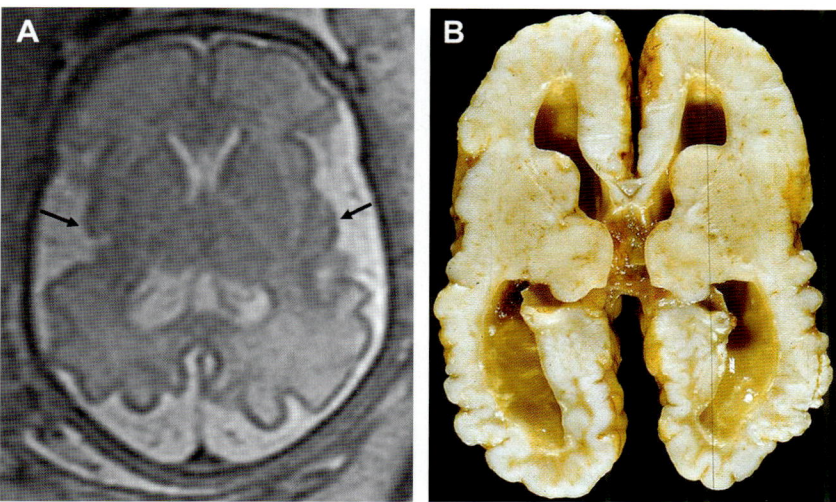

Fig. 8. Polymicrogyria. (A) Axial SS-FSE T2-weighted image of a 30-week EGA fetus demonstrates dysplastic-appearing sylvian fissures with multiple abnormal small infoldings of the cortex (arrows) consistent with perisylvian polymicrogyria. (B) Photograph of a gross specimen from a term infant with history of in utero CMV infection demonstrates numerous small irregular gyri consistent with polymicrogyria.

abnormalities of the cerebral and cerebellar white matter that are seen postnatally.[39] Associated eye anomalies, including subinal hemorrhages and microphthalmia, can occasionally be identified prenatally.[84]

CEPHALOCELES

Fetal MR imaging is valuable in the evaluation of cephaloceles because it can identify the portion of brain involved, and in older fetuses may even be able to identify involvement of the dural venous sinuses in cases of occipital and parietal encephaloceles. It is also capable of evaluating associated anomalies, such as anomalies of the corpus callosum, Chiari malformations, and cortical malformations. In the rare case of Chiari III malformations, in which there is a defect in the lower occipital bone and upper cervical spine, involvement of the brainstem and cerebellum can be assessed (Fig. 10).[85]

HOLOPROSENCEPHALY

Holoprosencephaly results from a failure of differentiation and cleavage of the prosencephalon. These can be the result of teratogens (maternal diabetes) and genetic factors (trisomy 13 and 18). These disorders all have in common some degree of callosal dysgenesis, along with absence of the septum pellucidum.[86] The holoprosencephalies represent a continuum and difficulty exists in determining a clear distinction between categories. Alobar holoprosencephaly is the most common form of holoprosencephaly identified on fetal ultrasound. It is easily assessed by fetal ultrasound, and the typical appearance is of a large monoventricle communicating with a dorsal cyst, fused thalami and basal ganglia, and a fused cortical mantle anteriorly without any interhemispheric fissure. No corpus callosum is identified in these patients. Because of the poor prognosis (most die shortly after birth or are stillborn) and easy identification of alobar holoprosencephaly by fetal ultrasound, other imaging studies are typically not performed. Semilobar and lobar holoprosencephalies are more difficult to detect on fetal ultrasound.[87] In semilobar holoprosencephaly, the interhemispheric fissure and falx cerebri are partially formed. There is still some degree of incomplete separation of the basal ganglia, and a third ventricle and incompletely formed lateral ventricles may be seen. Incomplete separation of the frontal lobes is still present, and only the splenium of the corpus callosum with or without a portion of the posterior body of the corpus callosum may be seen (Fig. 11). In lobar holoprosencephaly the ventricular system is further formed with identifiable frontal horns of the lateral ventricle, although they may be rudimentary. The degree of nonseparation of the forebrain is also mild, and in the mildest form only the hypothalamus is not separated. The body and splenium of the corpus callosum can be visualized.[88,89] Fetal MR imaging

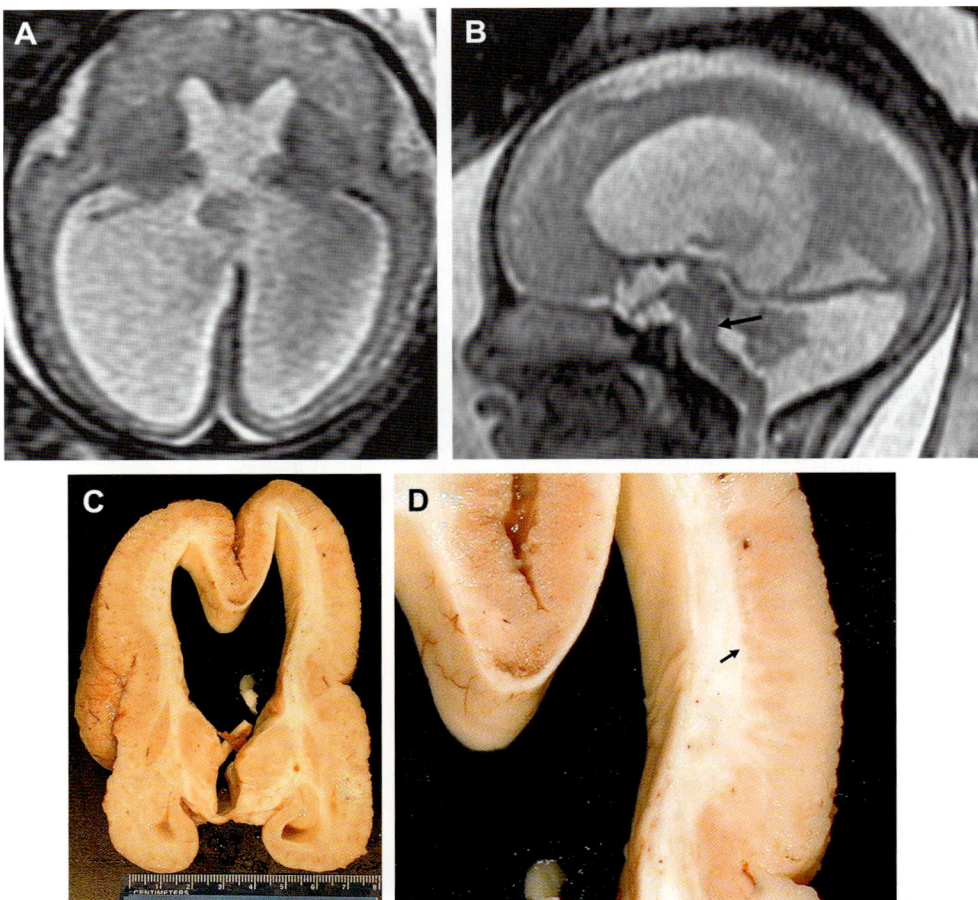

Fig. 9. Walker-Warburg syndrome. (*A*) Axial T2 SSFSE of a 31-week EGA fetus demonstrates ventriculomegaly. In addition, shallow, irregular sulci are noted. (*B*) Sagittal T2 SSFSE from the same fetus demonstrates a "kink" (*arrow*) at the pontomesencephalic junction and cerebellar vermian hypoplasia. (*C, D*) Photograph of a gross specimen (*C*) from a different patient who had Walker-Warburg syndrome demonstrates the abnormal appearance of the cortex and marked hydrocephalus. On the magnified image (*D*) irregular projections of cortex into the white matter can be seen (*arrow*).

can assess the degree of callosal development and separation of the frontal lobes and deep gray nuclei. In addition, associated anomalies of cortical development may be seen.

Associated eye and facial anomalies can be identified on fetal ultrasound and on fetal MR imaging. In alobar holoprosencephaly, severe midline facial deformities (cleft lip, cleft palate) are present because of absence or hypoplasia of the premaxillary segment of the face. In the extreme forms the orbits and globes fuse resulting in cyclopia. Facial abnormalities in semilobar holoprosencephaly are mild or absent.

Middle interhemispheric (MIH) variant, also known as syntelencephaly, is another form of holoprosencephaly. Unlike the classical holoprosencephaly, which is believed to be attributable to lack of expression of genes in the notochord or floor plate, MIH variant is believed to be the result of underexpression of genes involved in the development of the roof plate.[90] The result is a lack of induction of dorsal midline structures. There is fusion of the sylvian fissure across the midline with the posterior frontal and parietal lobes. The interhemispheric fissure is formed in the anterior frontal and in the occipital lobes. The callosal genu and the splenium are formed, but the body is absent.[90] Patients usually have mild to moderate cognitive impairment, mild visual impairment, and spasticity. Seizures may be seen in up to 40%, which is similar to the incidence in classic holoprosencephaly, but they do not demonstrate the endocrine dysfunction found in patients who have classic holoprosencephaly.[89] Distinguishing the MIH

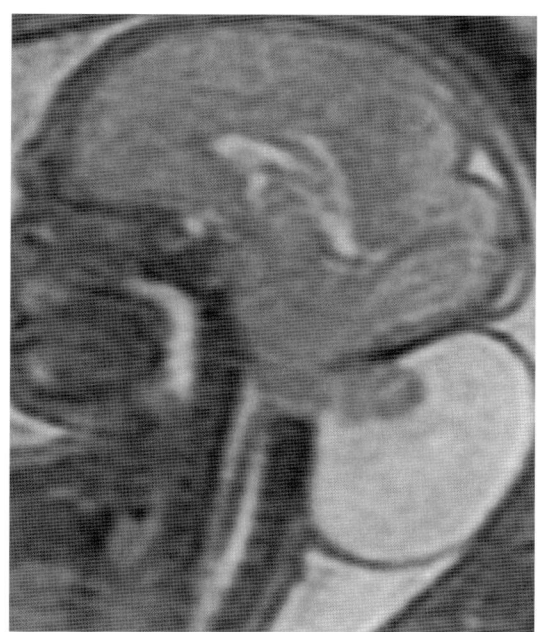

Fig. 10. Chiari III malformation. Sagittal SSFSE in a 23-week EGA fetus demonstrates a low occipital, high cervical bony defect through which neural tissue herniates into a cystic structure consistent with an encephalocele.

variant from other holoprosencephalies or midline migrational anomalies may be difficult by ultrasound, but is possible with fetal MR imaging.[91]

HEMORRHAGE AND VASCULAR MALFORMATIONS

Fetal MR imaging can be useful for the assessment of intracranial hemorrhage, and T1-weighted images and gradient echo T2-weighted images are beneficial in this regard. Hemorrhage is typically low in signal on T2 and high in signal on T1. Although the MR appearance of hemorrhage in children and adults typically depends on the age of the hemorrhage,[92] the signal patterns for evolving hemorrhage in the fetal brain are not well defined. Typically only one fetal MR is performed during gestation, and no complete studies have been performed. In addition, fetal hemoglobin has a higher affinity for oxygen, and the degradation process may be quicker in the fetus.[40]

Germinal matrix hemorrhages can be observed in the fetus. In term neonates, germinal matrix hemorrhage is associated with anoxia, acidosis, and changes in blood pressure associated with delivery. The pathophysiologic mechanisms of fetal germinal matrix hemorrhage are still unclear.[93,94] The detection of small germinal matrix hemorrhages is difficult because the germinal matrix has a similar signal to blood on both T1- and T2-weighted images. A T2*-weighted gradient image may be helpful to confirm blood, which may appear more hypointense than the germinal matrix.[95] These hemorrhages often originate from the anterior ganglionic eminence, which is a highly proliferative portion of the germinal matrix. Rupture of the ependyma in association with the germinal matrix hemorrhage leads to intraventricular hemorrhage (**Fig. 12**). Compression of medullary veins draining into the ventricular system by the hemorrhage can also lead to injury of the adjacent periventricular white matter with development of intraparenchymal hemorrhage A study by Morioka and colleagues[93] found that neurodevelopmental outcome in fetuses with germinal matrix hemorrhage depended on the presence and severity of parenchymal damage.

A potential cause of fetal intracranial hemorrhage is a vascular malformation. Dural arteriovenous fistulas are rare congenital malformations and are often located medially and posteriorly, and typically involve the torcula herophili.[95] On ultrasound, they typically appear as a heterogeneous mass posterior to the vermis and may contain a more hyperechoic nodule centrally.[95] Characteristic MR imaging findings consist of a dural-based mass centered at the torcula that demonstrates heterogeneous signal on T1-weighted images (**Fig. 13**).[95] On imaging follow-up the mass becomes more heterogeneous and concentric rings typical of thrombosis may be seen. Complications include hydrocephalus and infarction, and fetal MR imaging is beneficial for assessing for parenchymal injury.[96] Dural arteriovenous fistulas are considered to be associated with a poor neurologic outcome; however, favorable outcome has been reported when they thrombose in utero.[95,97,98] Malformations of the vein of Galen are also rare, and consist of abnormal connections occurring between intracranial arteries and the persistent median prosencephalic vein of Markowski. These malformations are visualized on ultrasound as a cyst-like structure in the region of the vein of Galen, and the vascular nature can be confirmed by Doppler. Vein of Galen malformation may result in a steal of blood flow from the surrounding brain parenchyma leading to ischemia (**Fig. 14**). The main differential diagnosis is an arteriovenous malformation (AVM) draining into the vein of Galen, and differentiating between the two is important because the outcomes can differ. The vein of Galen can be treated postnatally and have a good outcome, whereas an AVM typically has a worse prognosis.[99] Fetal MR imaging can be useful for identifying the exact nature of the

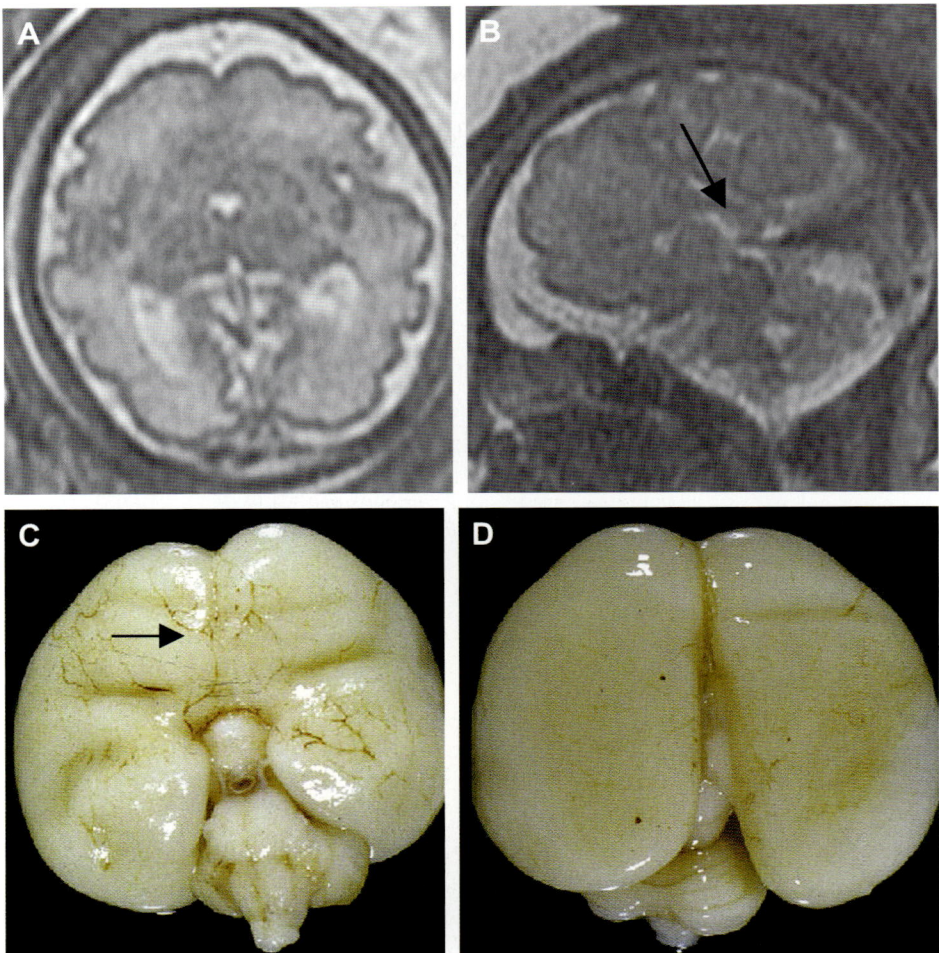

Fig. 11. Semilobar holoprosencephaly. (A) Axial T2 SSFSE in a 33-week EGA fetus demonstrates fusion of the cerebral hemispheres anteriorly. (B) Sagittal T2 SSFSE from the same fetus demonstrates formation of the splenium and posterior body of the corpus callosum (arrow). The anterior aspect of the corpus callosum is not formed. (C, D) Photographs of a gross specimen (C is ventral, D is dorsal view) from a 22-week fetus with semilobar holoprosencephaly from showing absence of the interhemispheric fissure anteriorly (C) but it is present posteriorly (D). The olfactory bulbs were also absent.

malformation and resultant intracranial complications, such as areas of encephalomalacia and hemorrhage.

VASCULAR INSULTS AND TWIN–TWIN TRANSFUSION

Monochorionic twins are at risk for developing ischemic parenchymal insults. The fetuses share the same placenta and there is increased likelihood of abnormal vascular connections resulting in abnormal blood flow to the fetuses. Twin–twin transfusion syndrome results when blood abnormally flows from one twin (donor) to the other recipient twin. The donor twin is smaller and develops oligohydramnios, the recipient twin develops volume overload and polyhydramnios, and both twins are at risk for cerebral ischemia. There is a 10-fold reported increased risk for the development of white matter injury in monochorionic twins compared with dichorionic twins (33% versus 3.3%).[100] Co-twin demise is another complication of monochorionic twin pregnancies, and is associated with a greater risk for neurologic impairment in the surviving twin (**Fig. 15**).[101] This impairment may result from thromboembolic events in the surviving twin or result from hypoperfusion.[101] Fetal MR imaging is valuable in assessing for regions of ischemic parenchymal injury, which appear as regions of increased T2 signal

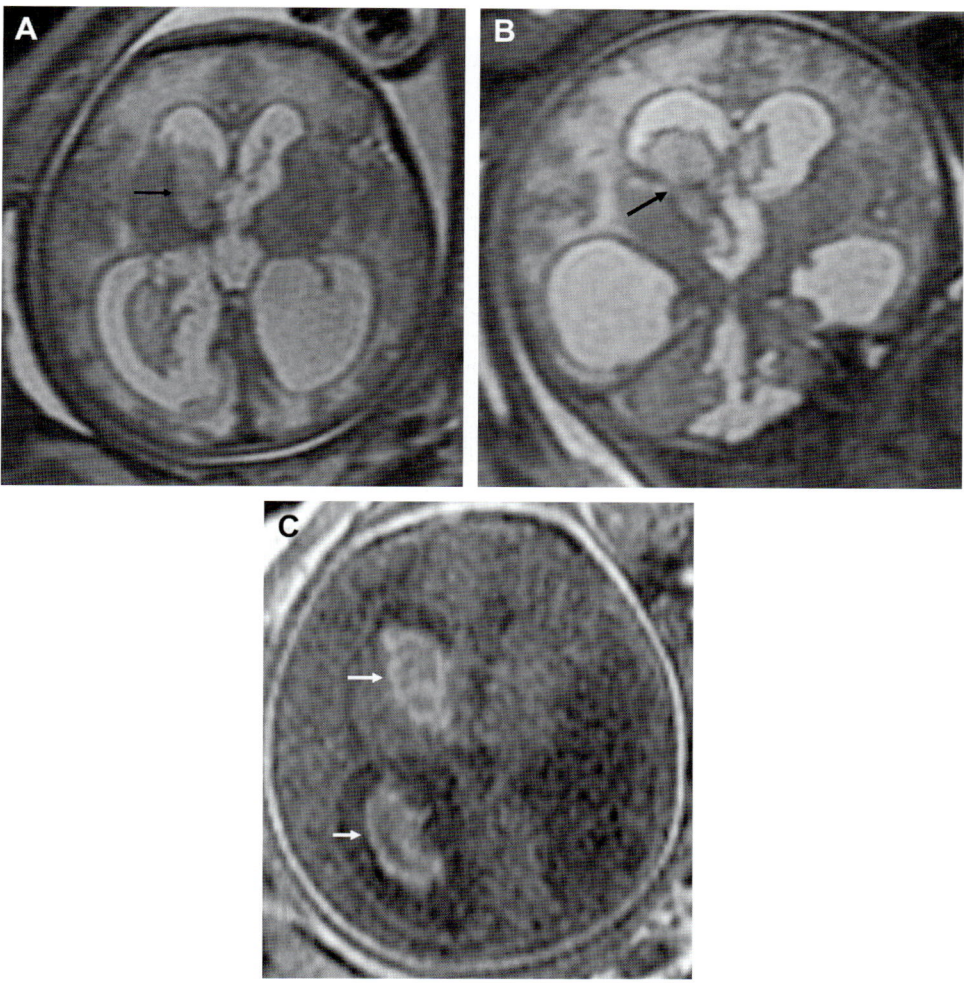

Fig. 12. Germinal matrix hemorrhage with rupture into the lateral ventricle. Axial (A) and coronal (B) T2 SSFSE of a 33-week EGA fetus with hemorrhage adjacent to the right caudothalamic notch (arrow). Intraventricular extension and hydrocephalus with diffuse edema and or injury are present. (C) Axial T1-weighted image from the same patient. The intraventricular hemorrhage demonstrates T1 hyperintense signal (arrows).

within the white matter, cerebral cortex, or germinal matrix.[23] The identification of such areas of encephalomalacia and periventricular white matter injury is important because they are associated with long-term neurodevelopmental deficits.[93] Diffusion-weighted MR imaging may lead to earlier detection of areas of ischemia in fetuses at risk for brain injury.[102]

Other causes of fetal ischemic insult include placental insufficiency, infectious causes, or maternal complications, including hypovolemic shock, abdominal trauma, hypoxia, hypertension, or drug use. Ischemic injuries have also been identified adjacent to mass lesions, such as neoplasms and subdural hematomas, and may result from compression. A study by Garel and colleagues[103] found that MR was a valuable tool in detecting the sequelae of ischemia involving the cortex, which was demonstrated by the presence of laminar necrosis or polymicrogyria and white matter lesions. Laminar necrosis and calcified leukomalacia are well demonstrated using T1-weighted sequences, and T2* imaging can be used to demonstrated regions of previous hemorrhage. In the future diffusion-tensor MR imaging may be of benefit in identifying the microstructural damage resulting from ischemic insult.[103]

ABNORMALITIES OF THE POSTERIOR FOSSA

Abnormalities of the posterior fossa are one of the most common findings on fetal imaging.[104]

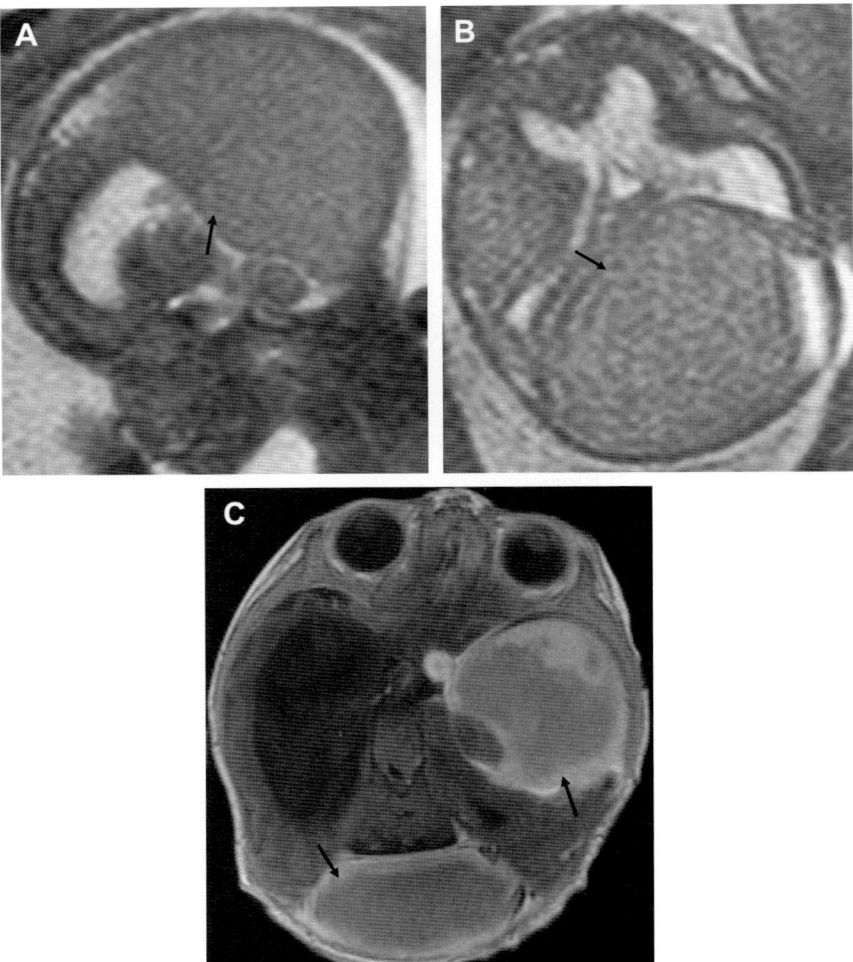

Fig. 13. Dural arteriovenous fistula. Sagittal (*A*) and axial (*B*) T2 SSFSE images of a 22-week EGA fetus demonstrate ventriculomegaly and an isointense, subdural mass within the posterior fossa (*arrow*). This mass was determined to be a hematoma, and was surgically evacuated shortly after birth. Abnormal vasculature consistent with a dural arteriovenous fistula was noted by the neurosurgeon. (*C*) Axial T1-weighted image obtained at 1 day of age demonstrates hematomas involving the posterior and middle cranial fossas (*arrows*).

Posterior fossa evaluation may be limited on ultrasound, especially in the third trimester secondary to ossification of the skull. Fetal MR imaging allows direct visualization of the posterior fossa structures, such as the vermis, cerebellar hemispheres, and brainstem. Posterior fossa abnormalities are heterogeneous and complex, and the evaluation of these anomalies by fetal MR imaging has been complicated by false-positive and false-negative diagnoses.[105–111]

One of the more common sonographic diagnoses is the Dandy-Walker complex, which is a continuum of posterior fossa cystic anomalies and consists of varying degrees of cerebellar or vermian hypoplasia, including the Dandy-Walker malformation, vermian hypoplasia, and mega cisterna magna (**Fig. 16**). Some authors use the term Dandy-Walker variant, which leads to confusion because some may use this to refer to a hypoplastic cerebellar vermis and a large cistern magna, whereas others may use it to refer to the Dandy-Walker malformation in which one or more of the fourth ventricular outflow foramina are patent. Because of the marked heterogeneity of brain abnormalities in both "Dandy Walker malformation" and "Dandy Walker variant," the effect of these abnormalities on neurodevelopmental outcome is poorly understood. Adopting a more descriptive approach of the findings as detected by either prenatal ultrasound or MR imaging (rather than classifying the abnormality into Dandy-Walker malformation or Dandy-Walker variant) will assist

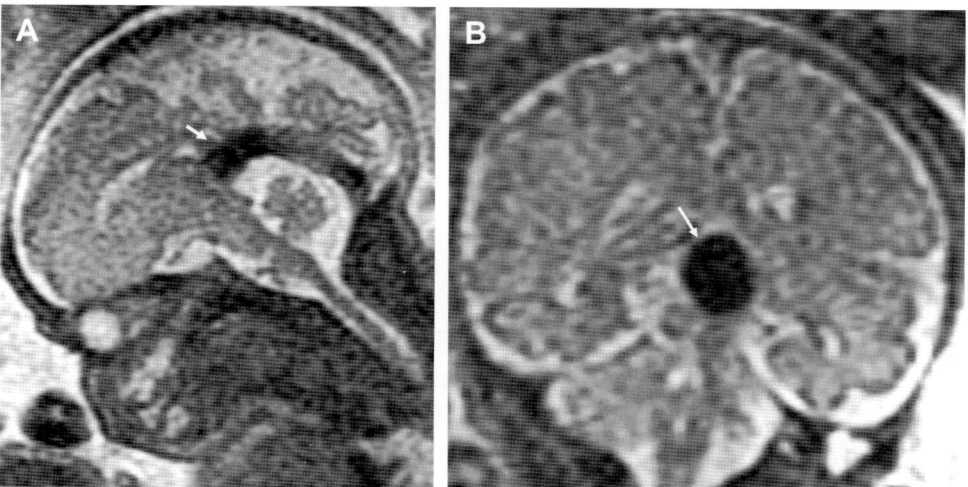

Fig. 14. Sagittal (A) and coronal (B) T2 SSFSE demonstrates a large flow void in the expected region of the vein of Galen (arrow) and continuing into the straight sinus.

in our eventual understanding of these complex abnormalities, their embryology, etiology, and neurodevelopmental outcome.

Hypoplasia or absence of the cerebellar vermis, hypoplasia of the cerebellar hemispheres, and enlargement of the posterior fossa and fourth ventricle have been classically described as the Dandy-Walker malformation. The enlargement of the posterior fossa results in an elevation of the torcula that is nicely demonstrated on the sagittal images, and is frequently associated with hypoplasia of the brainstem. Additional CNS anomalies, such as agenesis of the corpus callosum, holoprosencephaly, schizencephaly, and heterotopia, are associated with a worse prognosis[112–114] and are typically better evaluated by fetal MR imaging.

Vermian hypoplasia is a more subtle abnormality and is typically identified by incomplete covering of the fourth ventricle on ultrasound. Patients are often referred for fetal MR imaging to determine if the vermis is small or if there is a prominent cisterna magna. On fetal MR imaging, the vermis can be directly measured and the cerebellar hemispheres and brainstem can also be evaluated. In about one third of cases with presumed diagnosis

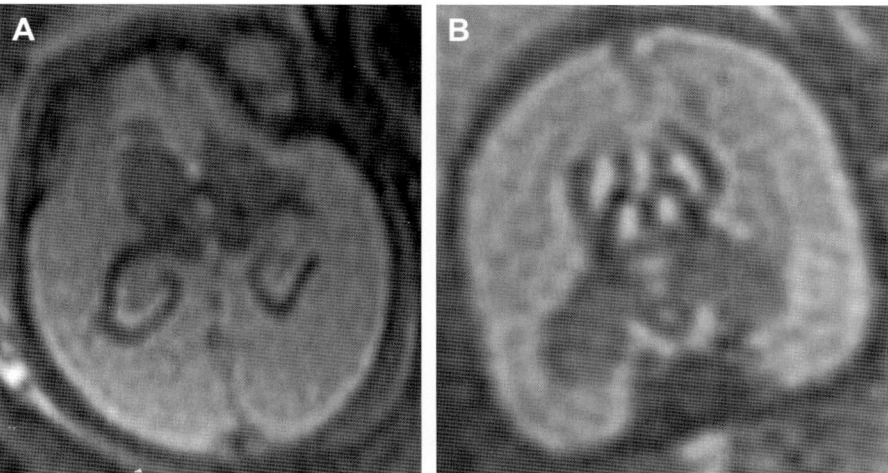

Fig. 15. Co-twin demise. Axial (A) and coronal (B) T2 SSFSE of a 25-week EGA fetus status post demise of the monochorionic twin. There is massive diffuse loss of supratentorial brain parenchyma. Periventricular low T2 signal is noted, which is consistent with either a hemorrhage or calcification.

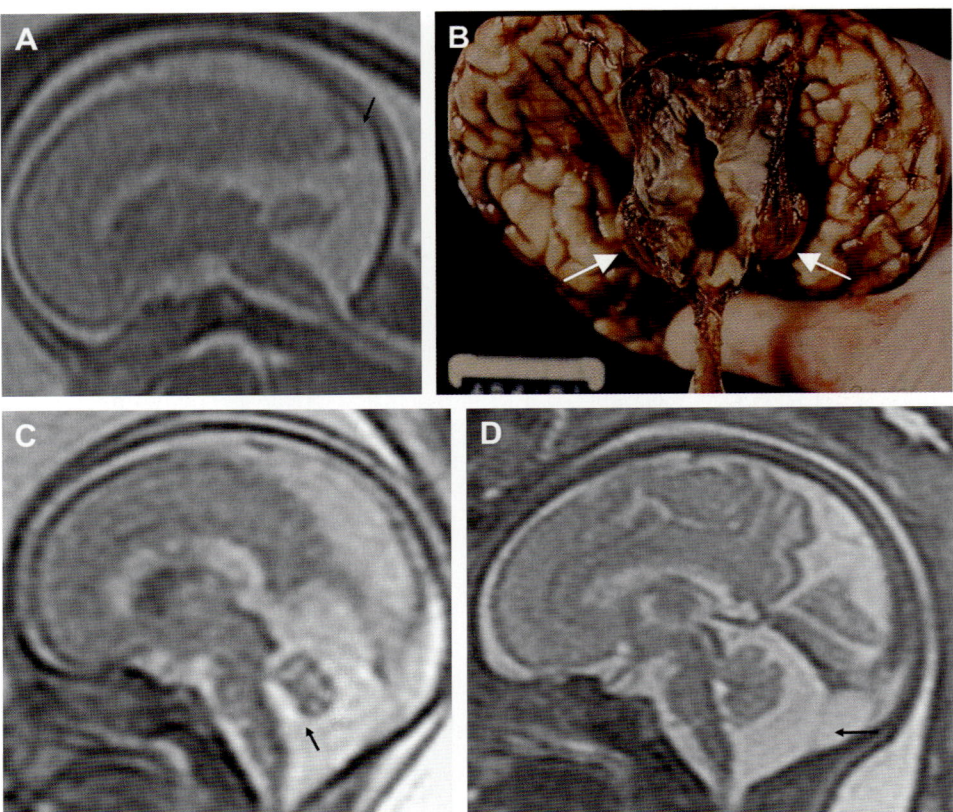

Fig. 16. Spectrum of posterior fossa anomalies. (A) Sagittal T2 SSFSE of a 23-week EGA fetus demonstrates vermian hypoplasia, enlargement of the posterior fossa, and elevation of the tentorium (arrow) consistent with Dandy-Walker malformation. (B) Photograph of a gross specimen of a different patient who had Dandy-Walker malformation demonstrates absence of the vermis and hypoplasia of the cerebellar hemispheres (arrows). (C) Sagittal T2 SSFSE of a 23-week EGA fetus demonstrates mild vermian hypoplasia demonstrated by a lack of complete coverage of the fourth ventricle (arrow). (D) Sagittal T2 SSFSE of a 29-week EGA fetus demonstrates a prominent posterior fossa fluid collection (arrow), but the vermis is normal in configuration and the tentorium is normally located, consistent with mega cisterna magna.

of inferior vermian hypoplasia on prenatal ultrasound and fetal MR imaging, the vermis appears normal on postnatal imaging.[104,105] This finding has important implications because some studies have shown neurodevelopmental abnormalities in children who have inferior vermian hypoplasia.[106]

Although rare, hemorrhage can occur within the cerebellum, and may result from infection, such as cytomegalovirus. The presence of cerebellar hemorrhage should, therefore, raise the suspicion of a congenital infection and a search for associated anomalies, such as intrauterine growth ardation, calcifications, and microcephaly, should be undertaken.[115,116] Other causes of cerebellar hemorrhage include immune and nonimmune hydrops, which may result from associated hematologic abnormalities.[117] Germinal matrix hemorrhage within the cerebellum may also occur.

Chiari II

Myelomeningoceles are one of the most common spinal anomalies detected on fetal ultrasound. They are almost always seen in associated with hindbrain malformation referred to as Chiari II, which consists of the findings of a small posterior fossa and herniation of the cerebellar tissue into the cervical subarachnoid space (**Fig. 17**). Chiari II malformations are easily assessed by fetal ultrasound, but fetal MR imaging has the benefit of assessing for other associated anomalies, such as callosal agenesis or hypogenesis,

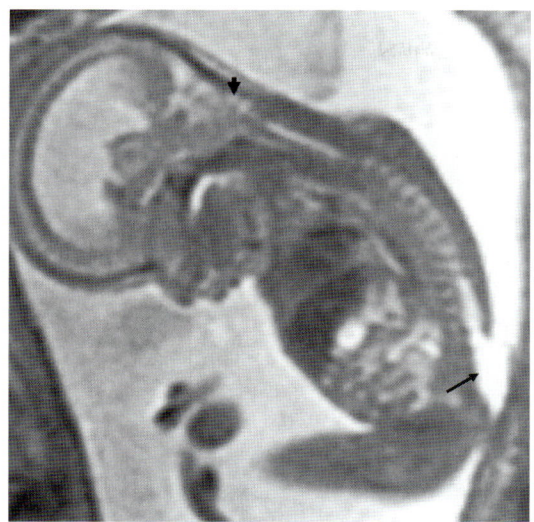

Fig. 17. Chiari II malformation. Sagittal T2 SSFSE image of a 22-week EGA fetus demonstrates a defect in the lumbosacral region (*thin arrow*) consistent with a myelomeningocele. A small posterior fossa is noted along with low-lying cerebellar tonsils (*thick arrow*) and marked ventriculomegaly.

cerebellar dysplasia, periventricular heterotopia, syringohydromyelia, and diastematomyelia.[23,118] Currently, several centers perform fetal surgery for repair of myelomeningoceles.[119]

CONGENITAL NEOPLASM

Intracranial neoplasms occurring during fetal life are rare, and account for approximately 0.5% to 1.9% of pediatric neoplasms.[120–122] The prognosis is typically poor, with postnatal survival reported around 28%.[123,124] Teratomas account for 50% and gliomas are the second most common (25%).[40] Other reported neoplasms include craniopharyngioma, hamartomas, choroid plexus papilloma, and hemangioblastoma.[125] Intracranial teratomas are heterogeneous in appearance. They are composed of solid and cystic components, and when the cystic component predominates they may be difficult to distinguish from an arachnoid cyst (**Fig. 18**). The imaging findings of glial neoplasms, craniopharyngiomas, and hamartomas are variable; however, craniopharyngiomas

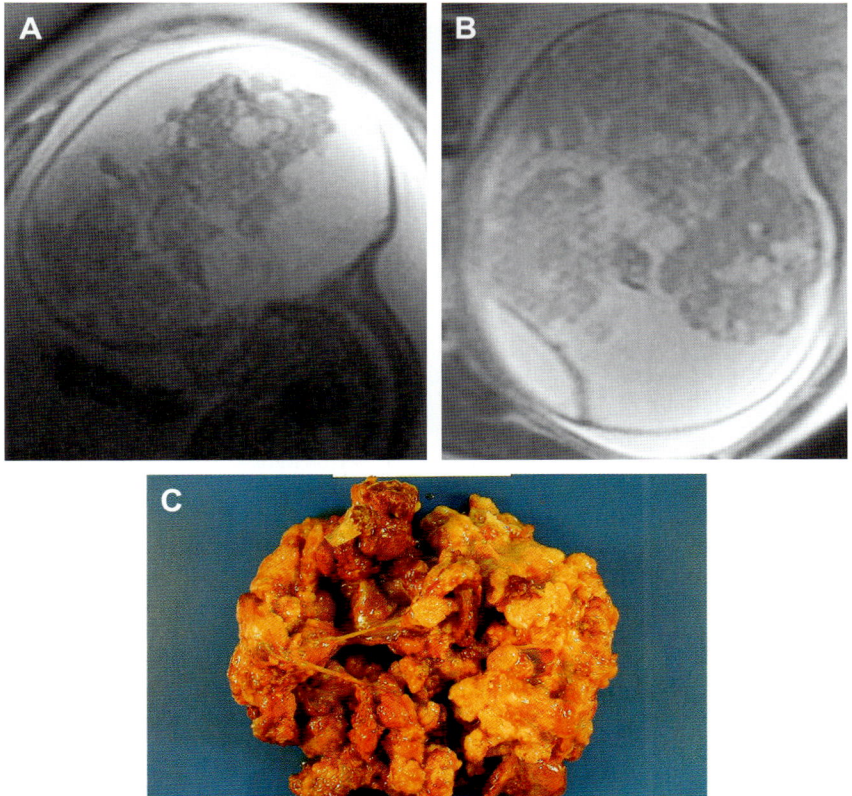

Fig. 18. Teratoma. Sagittal (*A*) and axial (*B*) T2 SSFSE in a 28-week EGA fetus demonstrates a large heterogeneous mass. No normal brain parenchyma is identified, and there is an enlarged head circumference. (*C*) Photograph of the gross specimen obtained at autopsy from the same patient demonstrates a multilobulated mass.

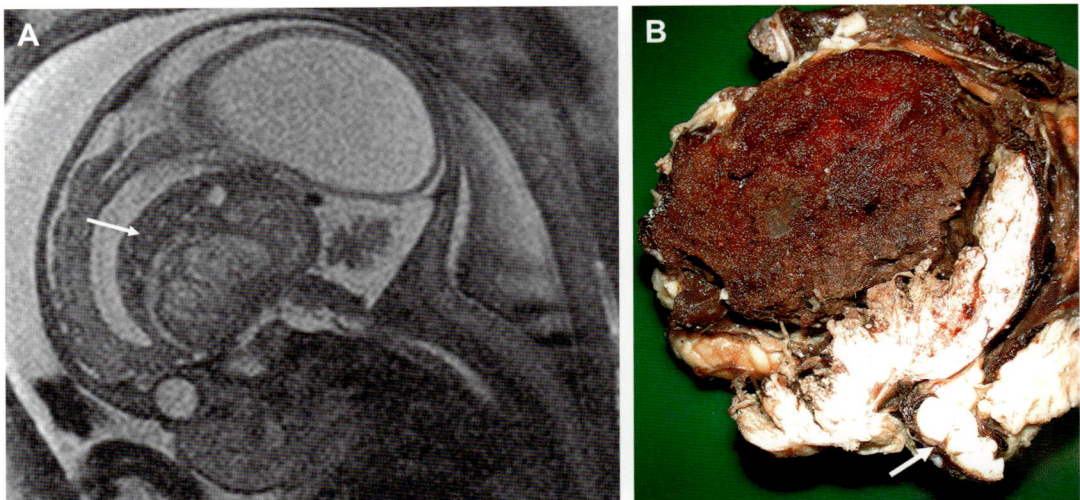

Fig. 19. Craniopharyngioma. (*A*) Sagittal T2 SSFSE in a 34-week EGA fetus demonstrates a midline heterogeneous mass in the suprasellar region (*arrow*). There is associated hydrocephalus. On autopsy, this was found to be a craniopharyngioma. (*B*) Photograph of gross specimen cut in the sagittal plane from the same patient demonstrates the large size of the lesion in comparison with the brain. The brainstem is visible in the lower aspect of the image (*arrow*).

tend to be located in the sellar region in the midline (**Fig. 19**). A study by Cassart and colleagues[125] found that fetal MR imaging was able to better determine the extent of tumoral extension than ultrasound, allowing them to assess the degree of involvement of adjacent structures, thus providing information concerning likelihood of surgical resection and prognosis.

CONGENITAL INFECTIONS

Various infections can involve the fetal nervous system, including the TORCH infections (toxoplasmosis, rubella, cytomegalovirus, and herpes simplex infections) and HIV, varicella, and acute maternal sepsis (typically group B streptococcus). The most common of these infections are cytomegalovirus and toxoplasmosis.[50,126–130] The effect of an infection of the fetal nervous system depends on the stage of development during which it occurs. Those infections occurring in the first two trimesters typically result in congenital malformations, whereas those occurring in the third trimester result in destructive lesions.[50] The findings of intrauterine growth retardation, intracranial and intrahepatic calcifications, ventriculomegaly, hyperechogenic bowel, or hydrops fetalis on ultrasound should raise the suspicion of fetal infection.[128] Intracranial hemorrhage has been reported as a complication of intracranial infections, especially in association with cytomegalovirus.[1] Other sequelae, such as cortical malformations, including lissencephaly and polymicrogyria, and delayed cortical maturation are well assessed on fetal MR imaging, and fetal MR imaging is an important adjunct to ultrasound when infection is suspected because it gives the best evaluation of the extent of parenchymal damage.[50]

SUMMARY

Fetal MR imaging provides a useful adjunct in the evaluation of anomalies of the fetal brain noted on ultrasound. The higher resolution of fetal MR imaging allows for improved assessment of cortical malformations and other anomalies. The use of fetal MR imaging is relatively new, however, and understanding of the imaging findings continues to evolve. In addition, the improvement of newer techniques, such as diffusion-weighted MR imaging, should lead to improved understanding of the developing fetal brain and the impact of ischemic, infectious, and developmental insults.

REFERENCES

1. Girard N, Raybaud C, Dercole C, et al. In vivo MRI of the fetal brain. Neuroradiology 1993;35(6): 431–6.
2. Brisse H, Fallet C, Sebag G, et al. Supratentorial parenchyma in the developing fetal brain: in vitro MR study with histologic comparison. AJNR Am J Neuroradiol 1997;18(8):1491–7.

3. Girard N, Raybaud C, Poncet M. In vivo MR study of brain maturation in normal fetuses. AJNR Am J Neuroradiol 1995;16(2):407–13.
4. Garel C, Chantrel E, Brisse H, et al. Fetal cerebral cortex: normal gestational landmarks identified using prenatal MR imaging. AJNR Am J Neuroradiol 2001;22(1):184–9.
5. Garel C, Chantrel E, Elmaleh M, et al. Fetal MRI: normal gestational landmarks for cerebral biometry, gyration and myelination. Childs Nerv Syst 2003; 19(7–8):422–5.
6. Levine D, Barnes PD, Madsen JR, et al. Central nervous system abnormalities assessed with prenatal magnetic resonance imaging. Obstet Gynecol 1999;94(6):1011–9.
7. Simon EM, Goldstein RB, Coakley FV, et al. Fast MR imaging of fetal CNS anomalies in utero. AJNR Am J Neuroradiol 2000;21(9):1688–98.
8. Levine D, Barnes PD, Madsen JR, et al. Fetal central nervous system anomalies: MR imaging augments sonographic diagnosis. Radiology 1997; 204(3):635–42.
9. Levine D, Barnes PD, Robertson RR, et al. Fast MR imaging of fetal central nervous system abnormalities. Radiology 2003;229(1):51–61.
10. Wagenvoort AM, Bekker MN, Go AT, et al. Ultrafast scan magnetic resonance in prenatal diagnosis. Fetal Diagn Ther 2000;15(6):364–72.
11. Glenn OA, Norton ME, Goldstein RB, et al. Prenatal diagnosis of polymicrogyria by fetal magnetic resonance imaging in monochorionic cotwin death. J Ultrasound Med 2005;24(5):711–6.
12. de Laveaucoupet J, Audibert F, Guis F, et al. Fetal magnetic resonance imaging (MRI) of ischemic brain injury. Prenat Diagn 2001;21(9):729–36.
13. Sonigo PC, Rypens FF, Carteret M, et al. MR imaging of fetal cerebral anomalies. Pediatr Radiol 1998;28(4):212–22.
14. Glenn OA, Goldstein RB, Li KC, et al. Fetal magnetic resonance imaging in the evaluation of fetuses referred for sonographically suspected abnormalities of the corpus callosum. J Ultrasound Med 2005;24(6):791–804.
15. Schneider JF, Confort-Gouny S, Le Fur Y, et al. Diffusion-weighted imaging in normal fetal brain maturation. Eur Radiol 2007;17(9):2422–9.
16. Kim DH, Chung S, Vigneron DB, et al. Diffusion-weighted imaging of the fetal brain in vivo. Magn Reson Med 2008;59(1):216–20.
17. Huang H, Zhang J, Wakana S, et al. White and gray matter development in human fetal, newborn and pediatric brains. Neuroimage 2006;33(1):27–38.
18. Gupta RK, Hasan KM, Trivedi R, et al. Diffusion tensor imaging of the developing human cerebrum. J Neurosci Res 2005;81(2):172–8.
19. Bui T, Daire JL, Chalard F, et al. Microstructural development of human brain assessed in utero by diffusion tensor imaging. Pediatr Radiol 2006; 36(11):1133–40.
20. Girard N, Gouny SC, Viola A, et al. Assessment of normal fetal brain maturation in utero by proton magnetic resonance spectroscopy. Magn Reson Med 2006;56(4):768–75.
21. Kok RD, van den Berg PP, van den Bergh AJ, et al. Maturation of the human fetal brain as observed by 1H MR spectroscopy. Magn Reson Med 2002; 48(4):611–6.
22. Kok RD, van den Bergh AJ, Heerschap A, et al. Metabolic information from the human fetal brain obtained with proton magnetic resonance spectroscopy. Am J Obstet Gynecol 2001;185(5): 1011–5.
23. Glenn OA, Barkovich J. Magnetic resonance imaging of the fetal brain and spine: an increasingly important tool in prenatal diagnosis: part 2. AJNR Am J Neuroradiol 2006;27(9):1807–14.
24. Jardri R, Pins D, Houfflin-Debarge V, et al. Fetal cortical activation to sound at 33 weeks of gestation: a functional MRI study. Neuroimage 2008;42(1): 10–8.
25. Moore RJ, Vadeyar S, Fulford J, et al. Antenatal determination of fetal brain activity in response to an acoustic stimulus using functional magnetic resonance imaging. Hum Brain Mapp 2001;12(2): 94–9.
26. Hykin J, Moore R, Duncan K, et al. Fetal brain activity demonstrated by functional magnetic resonance imaging. Lancet 1999;354(9179): 645–6.
27. Blaicher W, Prayer D, Bernaschek G. Magnetic resonance imaging and ultrasound in the assessment of the fetal central nervous system. J Perinat Med 2003;31(6):459–68.
28. Myers C, Duncan KR, Gowland PA, et al. Failure to detect intrauterine growth restriction following in utero exposure to MRI. Br J Radiol 1998;71(845): 549–51.
29. Clements H, Duncan KR, Fielding K, et al. Infants exposed to MRI in utero have a normal paediatric assessment at 9 months of age. Br J Radiol 2000; 73(866):190–4.
30. Kok RD, de Vries MM, Heerschap A, et al. Absence of harmful effects of magnetic resonance exposure at 1.5 T in utero during the third trimester of pregnancy: a follow-up study. Magn Reson Imaging 2004;22(6):851–4.
31. Yip YP, Capriotti C, Norbash SG, et al. Effects of MR exposure on cell proliferation and migration of chick motoneurons. J Magn Reson Imaging 1994; 4(6):799–804.
32. Yip YP, Capriotti C, Talagala SL, et al. Effects of MR exposure at 1.5 T on early embryonic development of the chick. J Magn Reson Imaging 1994;4(5): 742–8.

33. Yip YP, Capriotti C, Yip JW. Effects of MR exposure on axonal outgrowth in the sympathetic nervous system of the chick. J Magn Reson Imaging 1995;5(4):457–62.
34. Carnes KI, Magin RL. Effects of in utero exposure to 4.7 T MR imaging conditions on fetal growth and testicular development in the mouse. Magn Reson Imaging 1996;14(3):263–74.
35. Chew S, Ahmadi A, Goh PS, et al. The effects of 1.5T magnetic resonance imaging on early murine in-vitro embryo development. J Magn Reson Imaging 2001;13(3):417–20.
36. Kanal E, Borgstede JP, Barkovich AJ, et al. American College of Radiology white paper on MR safety. AJR Am J Roentgenol 2002;178(6):1335–47.
37. Shellock F, Kanal E. Bioeffects and safety of MR procedures. vol. 1. Philadelphia: WB Saunders; 1996.
38. De Santis M, Straface G, Cavaliere AF, et al. Gadolinium periconceptional exposure: pregnancy and neonatal outcome. Acta Obstet Gynecol Scand 2007;86(1):99–101.
39. Barkovich AJ. Pediatric neuroimaging. 3rd edition. Philadelphia: Lippincott Williams & Wilkins; 2005.
40. Garel C. MRI of the fetal brain: normal development and cerebral pathologies. Berlin: Springer; 2004.
41. Levine D, Barnes PD. Cortical maturation in normal and abnormal fetuses as assessed with prenatal MR imaging. Radiology 1999;210(3):751–8.
42. Kostovic I, Judas M, Rados M, et al. Laminar organization of the human fetal cerebrum revealed by histochemical markers and magnetic resonance imaging. Cereb Cortex 2002;12(5):536–44.
43. Fogliarini C, Chaumoitre K, Chapon F, et al. Assessment of cortical maturation with prenatal MRI: part II: abnormalities of cortical maturation. Eur Radiol 2005;15(9):1781–9.
44. Prayer D, Kasprian G, Krampl E, et al. MRI of normal fetal brain development. Eur J Radiol 2006;57(2):199–216.
45. Cohen-Sacher B, Lerman-Sagie T, Lev D, et al. Sonographic developmental milestones of the fetal cerebral cortex: a longitudinal study. Ultrasound Obstet Gynecol 2006;27(5):494–502.
46. Lan LM, Yamashita Y, Tang Y, et al. Normal fetal brain development: MR imaging with a half-Fourier rapid acquisition with relaxation enhancement sequence. Radiology 2000;215(1):205–10.
47. Bystron I, Blakemore C, Rakic P. Development of the human cerebral cortex: Boulder Committee revisited. Nat Rev Neurosci 2008;9(2):110–22.
48. Rutherford M, Jiang S, Allsop J, et al. MR imaging methods for assessing fetal brain development. Dev Neurobiol 2008;68(6):700–11.
49. Girard N, Raybaud C, Gambarelli D, et al. Fetal brain MR imaging. Magn Reson Imaging Clin N Am 2001;9(1):19–56, vii.
50. Barkovich AJ, Girard N. Fetal brain infections. Childs Nerv Syst 2003;19(7–8):501–7.
51. Brunel H, Girard N, Confort-Gouny S, et al. Fetal brain injury. J Neuroradiol 2004;31(2):123–37.
52. Cardoza JD, Goldstein RB, Filly RA. Exclusion of fetal ventriculomegaly with a single measurement: the width of the lateral ventricular atrium. Radiology 1988;169(3):711–4.
53. Goldstein RB, La Pidus AS, Filly RA, et al. Mild lateral cerebral ventricular dilatation in utero: clinical significance and prognosis. Radiology 1990;176(1):237–42.
54. Levine D, Trop I, Mehta TS, et al. MR imaging appearance of fetal cerebral ventricular morphology. Radiology 2002;223(3):652–60.
55. Garel C, Alberti C. Coronal measurement of the fetal lateral ventricles: comparison between ultrasonography and magnetic resonance imaging. Ultrasound Obstet Gynecol 2006;27(1):23–7.
56. Patel MD, Filly AL, Hersh DR, et al. Isolated mild fetal cerebral ventriculomegaly: clinical course and outcome. Radiology 1994;192(3):759–64.
57. Bromley B, Frigoletto FD Jr, Benacerraf BR. Mild fetal lateral cerebral ventriculomegaly: clinical course and outcome. Am J Obstet Gynecol 1991;164(3):863–7.
58. Gupta JK, Bryce FC, Lilford RJ. Management of apparently isolated fetal ventriculomegaly. Obstet Gynecol Surv 1994;49(10):716–21.
59. Gaglioti P, Danelon D, Bontempo S, et al. Fetal cerebral ventriculomegaly: outcome in 176 cases. Ultrasound Obstet Gynecol 2005;25(4):372–7.
60. Pilu G, Falco P, Gabrielli S, et al. The clinical significance of fetal isolated cerebral borderline ventriculomegaly: report of 31 cases and review of the literature. Ultrasound Obstet Gynecol 1999;14(5):320–6.
61. Mercier A, Eurin D, Mercier PY, et al. Isolated mild fetal cerebral ventriculomegaly: a retrospective analysis of 26 cases. Prenat Diagn 2001;21(7):589–95.
62. Vergani P, Locatelli A, Strobelt N, et al. Clinical outcome of mild fetal ventriculomegaly. Am J Obstet Gynecol 1998;178(2):218–22.
63. Falip C, Blanc N, Maes E, et al. Postnatal clinical and imaging follow-up of infants with prenatal isolated mild ventriculomegaly: a series of 101 cases. Pediatr Radiol 2007;37(10):981–9.
64. Mahony BS, Nyberg DA, Hirsch JH, et al. Mild idiopathic lateral cerebral ventricular dilatation in utero: sonographic evaluation. Radiology 1988;169(3):715–21.
65. Coakley FV, Hricak H, Filly RA, et al. Complex fetal disorders: effect of MR imaging on management–preliminary clinical experience. Radiology 1999;213(3):691–6.

66. Twining P, Jaspan T, Zuccollo J. The outcome of fetal ventriculomegaly. Br J Radiol 1994;67(793): 26–31.
67. Bertino RE, Nyberg DA, Cyr DR, et al. Prenatal diagnosis of agenesis of the corpus callosum. J Ultrasound Med 1988;7(5):251–60.
68. Callen PW, Callen AL, Glenn OA, et al. Columns of the fornix, not to be mistaken for the cavum septi pellucidi on prenatal sonography. J Ultrasound Med 2008;27(1):25–31.
69. Moutard ML, Kieffer V, Feingold J, et al. Agenesis of corpus callosum: prenatal diagnosis and prognosis. Childs Nerv Syst 2003;19(7-8):471–6.
70. d'Ercole C, Girard N, Cravello L, et al. Prenatal diagnosis of fetal corpus callosum agenesis by ultrasonography and magnetic resonance imaging. Prenat Diagn 1998;18(3):247–53.
71. Hetts SW, Sherr EH, Chao S, et al. Anomalies of the corpus callosum: an MR analysis of the phenotypic spectrum of associated malformations. AJR Am J Roentgenol 2006;187(5):1343–8.
72. Gupta JK, Lilford RJ. Assessment and management of fetal agenesis of the corpus callosum. Prenat Diagn 1995;15(4):301–12.
73. Barkovich AJ, Norman D. Anomalies of the corpus callosum: correlation with further anomalies of the brain. AJR Am J Roentgenol 1988; 151(1):171–9.
74. Blum A, Andre M, Droulle P, et al. Prenatal echographic diagnosis of corpus callosum agenesis. The Nancy experience 1982–1989. Genet Couns 1990;1(2):115–26.
75. Urbach H, Scheffler B, Heinrichsmeier T, et al. Focal cortical dysplasia of Taylor's balloon cell type: a clinicopathological entity with characteristic neuroimaging and histopathological features, and favorable postsurgical outcome. Epilepsia 2002; 43(1):33–40.
76. Quek SC, Yip W, Quek ST, et al. Cardiac manifestations in tuberous sclerosis: a 10-year review. J Paediatr Child Health 1998;34(3):283–7.
77. Webb DW, Thomas RD, Osborne JP. Cardiac rhabdomyomas and their association with tuberous sclerosis. Arch Dis Child 1993;68(3):367–70.
78. Merello E, Swanson E, De Marco P, et al. No major role for the EMX2 gene in schizencephaly. Am J Med Genet A 2008;146(9):1142–50.
79. Jansen A, Andermann E. Genetics of the polymicrogyria syndromes. J Med Genet 2005;42(5): 369–78.
80. Guerra MP, Cavalleri F, Migone N, et al. Intractable epilepsy in hemimegalencephaly and tuberous sclerosis complex. J Child Neurol 2007;22(1):80–4.
81. Billette de Villemeur T, Chiron C, Robain C. Unlayered polymicrogyria and agenesis of the corpus callosum: a relevant association? Acta Neuropathol 1992;83(3):265–70.
82. Barkovich AJ. Neuroimaging manifestations and classification of congenital muscular dystrophies. AJNR Am J Neuroradiol 1998;19(8):1389–96.
83. Monteagudo A, Alayon A, Mayberry P. Walker-Warburg syndrome: case report and review of the literature. J Ultrasound Med 2001;20(4):419–26.
84. Vainzof M, Richard P, Herrmann R, et al. Prenatal diagnosis in laminin alpha2 chain (merosin)-deficient congenital muscular dystrophy: a collective experience of five international centers. Neuromuscul Disord 2005;15(9–10):588–94.
85. Smith AB, Gupta N, Otto C, et al. Diagnosis of Chiari III malformation by second trimester fetal MRI with postnatal MRI and CT correlation. Pediatr Radiol 2007;37(10):1035–8.
86. Barkovich AJ. Apparent atypical callosal dysgenesis: analysis of MR findings in six cases and their relationship to holoprosencephaly. AJNR Am J Neuroradiol 1990;11(2):333–9.
87. Aubry MC, Aubry JP, Dommergues M. Sonographic prenatal diagnosis of central nervous system abnormalities. Childs Nerv Syst 2003;19(7–8): 391–402.
88. Oba H, Barkovich AJ. Holoprosencephaly: an analysis of callosal formation and its relation to development of the interhemispheric fissure. AJNR Am J Neuroradiol 1995;16(3):453–60.
89. Lewis AJ, Simon EM, Barkovich AJ, et al. Middle interhemispheric variant of holoprosencephaly: a distinct cliniconeuroradiologic subtype. Neurology 2002;59(12):1860–5.
90. Simon EM, Hevner RF, Pinter JD, et al. The middle interhemispheric variant of holoprosencephaly. AJNR Am J Neuroradiol 2002;23(1):151–6.
91. Pulitzer SB, Simon EM, Crombleholme TM, et al. Prenatal MR findings of the middle interhemispheric variant of holoprosencephaly. AJNR Am J Neuroradiol 2004;25(6):1034–6.
92. Osborn AG. Diagnostic imaging. Brain. 1st edition. Salt Lake City (UT): Amirsys; 2004.
93. Morioka T, Hashiguchi K, Nagata S, et al. Fetal germinal matrix and intraventricular hemorrhage. Pediatr Neurosurg 2006;42(6):354–61.
94. Vergani P, Strobelt N, Locatelli A, et al. Clinical significance of fetal intracranial hemorrhage. Am J Obstet Gynecol 1996;175(3 Pt 1):536–43.
95. Glenn OA, Barkovich AJ. Magnetic resonance imaging of the fetal brain and spine: an increasingly important tool in prenatal diagnosis, part 1. AJNR Am J Neuroradiol 2006;27(8):1604–11.
96. Merzoug V, Flunker S, Drissi C, et al. Dural sinus malformation (DSM) in fetuses. Diagnostic value of prenatal MRI and follow-up. Eur Radiol 2008; 18(4):692–9.
97. Morita A, Meyer FB, Nichols DA, et al. Childhood dural arteriovenous fistulae of the posterior dural sinuses: three case reports and literature review.

Neurosurgery 1995;37(6):1193–9 [discussion: 1199–200].
98. Gicquel JM, Potier A, Sitruk S, et al. Normal outcome after prenatal diagnosis of thrombosis of the torcular Herophili. Prenat Diagn 2000;20(10): 824–7.
99. Brunelle F. Brain vascular malformations in the fetus: diagnosis and prognosis. Childs Nerv Syst 2003;19(7–8):524–8.
100. Bejar R, Vigliocco G, Gramajo H, et al. Antenatal origin of neurologic damage in newborn infants. II. Multiple gestations. Am J Obstet Gynecol 1990;162(5):1230–6.
101. van Heteren CF, Nijhuis JG, Semmekrot BA, et al. Risk for surviving twin after fetal death of co-twin in twin-twin transfusion syndrome. Obstet Gynecol 1998;92(2):215–9.
102. Garel C. New advances in fetal MR neuroimaging. Pediatr Radiol 2006;36(7):621–5.
103. Garel C, Delezoide AL, Elmaleh-Berges M, et al. Contribution of fetal MR imaging in the evaluation of cerebral ischemic lesions. AJNR Am J Neuroradiol 2004;25(9):1563–8.
104. Limperopoulos C, Robertson RL, Estroff JA, et al. Diagnosis of inferior vermian hypoplasia by fetal magnetic resonance imaging: potential pitfalls and neurodevelopmental outcome. Am J Obstet Gynecol 2006;194(4):1070–6.
105. Limperopoulos C, Robertson RL, Khwaja O, et al. How accurately does current fetal imaging identify posterior fossa abnormalities. Am J Roentgenol 2008;190:1637–43.
106. Siebert JR. A pathological approach to anomalies of the posterior fossa. Birth Defects Res A Clin Mol Teratol 2006;76(9):674–84.
107. Wald M, Lawrenz K, Deutinger J, et al. Verification of anomalies of the central nervous system detected by prenatal ultrasound. Ultraschall Med 2004;25(3):214–7.
108. Carroll SG, Porter H, Abdel-Fattah S, et al. Correlation of prenatal ultrasound diagnosis and pathologic findings in fetal brain abnormalities. Ultrasound Obstet Gynecol 2000;16(2):149–53.
109. Chang MC, Russell SA, Callen PW, et al. Sonographic detection of inferior vermian agenesis in Dandy-Walker malformations: prognostic implications. Radiology 1994;193(3):765–70.
110. Laing FC, Frates MC, Brown DL, et al. Sonography of the fetal posterior fossa: false appearance of mega-cisterna magna and Dandy-Walker variant. Radiology 1994;192(1):247–51.
111. Estroff JA, Scott MR, Benacerraf BR. Dandy-Walker variant: prenatal sonographic features and clinical outcome. Radiology 1992;185(3):755–8.
112. Golden JA, Rorke LB, Bruce DA. Dandy-Walker syndrome and associated anomalies. Pediatr Neurosci 1987;13(1):38–44.
113. Maria BL, Zinreich SJ, Carson BC, et al. Dandy-Walker syndrome revisited. Pediatr Neurosci 1987;13(1):45–51.
114. Bindal AK, Storrs BB, McLone DG. Management of the Dandy-Walker syndrome. Pediatr Neurosurg 1990;16(3):163–9.
115. Ortiz JU, Ostermayer E, Fischer T, et al. Severe fetal cytomegalovirus infection associated with cerebellar hemorrhage. Ultrasound Obstet Gynecol 2004;23(4):402–6.
116. Glenn OA, Bianco K, Barkovich AJ, et al. Fetal cerebellar hemorrhage in parvovirus-associated non-immune hydrops fetalis. J Matern Fetal Neonatal Med 2007;20(10):769–72.
117. Ghi T, Brondelli L, Simonazzi G, et al. Sonographic demonstration of brain injury in fetuses with severe red blood cell alloimmunization undergoing intrauterine transfusions. Ultrasound Obstet Gynecol 2004;23(5):428–31.
118. Wolpert SM, Anderson M, Scott RM, et al. Chiari II malformation: MR imaging evaluation. AJR Am J Roentgenol 1987;149(5):1033–42.
119. Fichter MA, Dornseifer U, Henke J, et al. Fetal spina bifida—current trends and prospects of intrauterine Neurosurgery. Fetal Diagn Ther 2008;23(4):271–86.
120. Buetow PC, Smirniotopoulos JG, Done S. Congenital brain tumors: a review of 45 cases. AJR Am J Roentgenol 1990;155(3):587–93.
121. Rickert CH. Neuropathology and prognosis of foetal brain tumours. Acta Neuropathol 1999;98(6): 567–76.
122. Cavalheiro S, Moron AF, Hisaba W, et al. Fetal brain tumors. Childs Nerv Syst 2003;19(7–8):529–36.
123. Isaacs H Jr. I. Perinatal brain tumors: a review of 250 cases. Pediatr Neurol 2002;27(4):249–61.
124. Isaacs H Jr. II. Perinatal brain tumors: a review of 250 cases. Pediatr Neurol 2002;27(5):333–42.
125. Cassart M, Bosson N, Garel C, et al. Fetal intracranial tumors: a review of 27 cases. Eur Radiol 2008; 18:2060–6.
126. Hollier LM, Grissom H. Human herpes viruses in pregnancy: cytomegalovirus, Epstein-Barr virus, and varicella zoster virus. Clin Perinatol 2005; 32(3):671–96.
127. Daniel Y, Gull I, Peyser MR, et al. Congenital cytomegalovirus infection. Eur J Obstet Gynecol Reprod Biol 1995;63(1):7–16.
128. Lipitz S, Yagel S, Shalev E, et al. Prenatal diagnosis of fetal primary cytomegalovirus infection. Obstet Gynecol 1997;89(5 Pt 1):763–7.
129. Dammann O, Leviton A. Maternal intrauterine infection, cytokines, and brain damage in the perm newborn. Pediatr Res 1997;42(1):1–8.
130. Dammann O, Leviton A. Infection remote from the brain, neonatal white matter damage, and cerebral palsy in the preterm infant. Semin Pediatr Neurol 1998;5(3):190–201.

Ultrasound of the Fetal Cranium: Review of Current Literature

Eyal Sheiner, MD, PhD[a], Jacques S. Abramowicz, MD[b],*

KEYWORDS

- Fetal cranium • Fetal anatomy • Ultrasound
- Craniosynostosis • Neural tube defects

Among the core goals of the prenatal ultrasound examination is characterization of the fetal organs as anatomically normal or abnormal. Deviations from normal require detailed specialized examination. Anomalies of the fetal brain are relatively common and have the potential to result in severe morbidity or mortality. Although much has been published regarding the fetal brain, less has been discussed about the skull. This article discusses normal and abnormal fetal skull anatomy as observed using ultrasound technology.

NORMAL SKULL AND SHAPE VARIATIONS

The skull bones are formed from mesenchymal condensations that develop into connective tissue and subsequently ossify (ie, membranous ossification).[1] Prenatal ultrasound study is able to depict ossified portions of the fetal skeleton as early as the late first trimester.[2] Ossified bones appear echogenic compared with hypoechoic cartilage.

Images of the skull are routinely obtained during ultrasound examination. The frontal, parietal, thin squama of the temporal bones, and occipital bones, which together form the calvaria, should be visualized. The cartilaginous zones of articulation of these bones, the coronal, sagittal, and lamboid sutures, are visible, along with the fontanelles, mainly the anterior and posterior (**Fig. 1**).[3,4]

The biparietal diameter (BPD) was the first reported related sonographic fetal measurement[5] and is considered a relatively accurate parameter for gestational age determination between 14 and 26 weeks of gestation, with variation of plus or minus 7 to10 days. The BPD is preferably measured on the transverse plane, from the outer edge of the proximal skull to the inner edge of the distal skull. The BPD is measured at the widest area on the skull and demonstrates the thalamic nuclei and the cavum septi pellucidi. The occipitofrontal diameter is measured from mid-echo to mid-echo (ie, the anteroposterior measurement obtained from outer skull to outer skull, excluding the skin). The cephalic index is the ratio of the biparietal to occipitofrontal diameters reported as a percentage (short axis/long axis $\times$ 100). Normal intrauterine cephalic index is 80%. The head circumference (HC) should always be measured, because most of the time it better reflects gestational age. This measurement is done either through tracing with digital calipers or calculation from the above two diameters. The cranium is considered to be brachycephalic (from the Greek *brachys*, meaning short) if the cephalic index is greater than 85% (ie, the head shape is rounded because the BPD is relatively large, whereas the occipitofrontal diameter is somewhat short) (**Fig. 2**), and dolichocephalic (from the Greek *dolikhos*, meaning long and thin, also known as scaphocephaly or boat-shape [Greek: *scaphe*]) if less than 75% (ie, the head shape is elongated).[6,7] Dolichocephaly is more common in preterm fetuses presenting as breech and more common in fetuses who have oligohydramnios of long-standing duration.[8] From 14 to 40 weeks'

---

[a] Department of Obstetrics & Gynecology, Soroka University Medical Center, Ben Gurion University of the Negev, Beer Sheva, Israel
[b] Department of Obstetrics & Gynecology, Rush University Medical Center, 1653 W Congress Parkway, Chicago, IL 60612, USA
* Corresponding author.
E-mail address: jacques_abramowicz@rush.edu (J.S. Abramowicz).

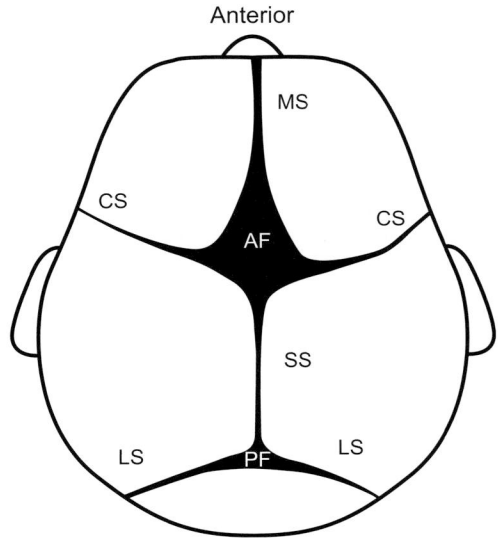

Fig. 1. Fetal cranium sutures and fontanelles. AF, anterior fontanelle; CS, coronal suture; LS, lambdoidal suture; MS, metopic suture; PF, posterior fontanelle; SS, sagittal suture.

gestation, there is no significant change in the cephalic index with gestational age.[9]

Variations in the shape of the fetal skull (eg, dolichocephaly, brachycephaly) may adversely affect the accuracy of the BPD measurement in estimating fetal age.[9,10] Controversy exists regarding the association between variation in shape and chromosomal abnormalities. Although Borenstein and colleagues[7] found an association between brachycephaly and trisomy 21 at 11 plus 0/7 to 13 plus 6/7 weeks of gestation, such association was not confirmed by others.[11] Borrell and colleagues[11] determined the cephalic index in 555 consecutive chromosomally normal fetuses and in 38 chromosomally abnormal fetuses before amniocentesis. A cephalic index greater than 0.85 was observed in 14% of fetuses who had Down syndrome and in 11% of normal fetuses. The authors concluded that brachycephaly is not a useful marker for Down syndrome in early midtrimester fetuses. Preliminary experience indicates that a cephalic index greater than 1 SD from the mean (less than 74% or greater than 83%) may be associated with significant alteration of the BPD measurement expected for a given gestational age, and therefore the head circumference can be used effectively as an alternative and more accurate means of establishing gestational age.[9]

Fetal head measurements can be correlated with the abdominal circumference (AC) or the femur length (FL). The normal head circumference/abdominal circumference ratio (HC/AC) is gestational age dependent and ranges between 1.07 and 1.26.[12] Alterations in this ratio may suggest a cranial anomaly. The normal femur length/biparietal diameter ratio (FL/BPD) is 0.71 to 0.87. This ratio may be altered when there is a change in either of these measurements.[12] Fetuses affected with Down syndrome demonstrate normal biparietal diameter (BPD), but high BPD/FL ratio, secondary to shortened femur length.[13]

The association between the second-trimester fetal biparietal diameter/nasal bone length (BPD/NBL) ratio and trisomy 21 was previously evaluated.[14] Thirty-one cases of trisomy 21 were compared with 136 matched euploid fetuses for maternal age, indication for referral, and gestational age. The mean NBL was shorter (mean ± SD, 2.3 ± 1.7 mm versus 3.9 ± 1.2 mm; $P<.001$) and the BPD/NBL ratio was greater (17.7 [range, 6.2–114] versus 11.7 [range, 5.8–80]; $P<.001$) for fetuses who had trisomy 21. The risk for trisomy 21 increased 2.4-fold (95% CI, 1.7–3.4) with every 1-mm decrease in NBL and increased 1.08-fold (95% CI, 1.03–1.12) with each unit increase in the BPD/NBL ratio ($P<.001$). The BPD/NBL ratio was found to be an independent predictor of trisomy 21 (odds ratio, 1.08; 95% CI, 1.03–1.11) in a multiple logistic regression model. The authors concluded that second-trimester BPD/NBL ratio was a significant and independent predictor of trisomy 21. An assessment of the BPD/NBL ratio may improve the detection rate of trisomy 21 cases when incorporated with current prenatal sonographic and maternal serum screening protocol.[14]

Head size should be carefully measured relative to the established gestational age, to determine the appropriateness of head size or the presence of micro- or macrocephaly. The shape of the

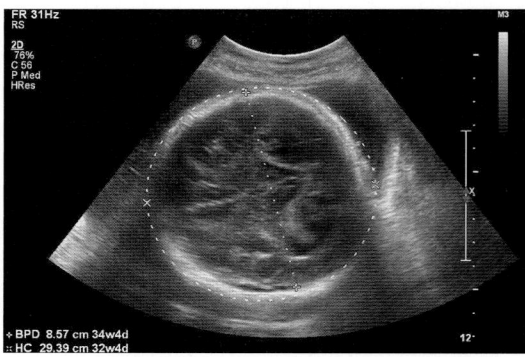

Fig. 2. Severe brachycephaly. Note that the BPD is consistent with a gestational age of 34 and 4/7 weeks in a 32-week fetus.

head should be evaluated also. Anomalies of the skull have been observed using ultrasound study during the early second trimester.[15] Ossification centers become visible near the end of the first trimester. At 16 weeks a three-dimensional (3D) sagittal scan displays the cranium and the echo-free fontanels and the cranial sutures (**Fig. 3**).[16] On an axial sonogram at the beginning of the second trimester, the head should be oval. The optimal time for viewing the cranial sutures is between 14 weeks and 16 weeks, and the earliest described cranial changes included abnormalities in biparietal distance.[17,18]

ABNORMAL SKULL
Craniosynostosis

Craniosynostosis is the premature fusion of a single or multiple cranial sutures.[12] It may occur either prenatally or perinatally.[19] This premature fusion restricts and distorts the growth of the skull, often resulting in increased intracranial pressure. The final abnormal skull shape depends on the specific suture fused and whether unilateral or bilateral sutures are involved.[20]

- Premature fusion of the coronal sutures compels the skull to grow wide relative to its length, resulting in brachycephaly.
- Premature fusion of the sagittal suture forces the skull to grow long relative to its width, resulting in dolichocephaly.
- Premature fusion of the metopic suture results in a narrow, triangular forehead with concavity of the temples, known as trigonocephaly.
- Premature fusion of either the coronal or lambdoid sutures results in asymmetrical, flat skull shape or plagiocephaly ("oblique" skull).
- Premature fusion of both the coronal and sagittal sutures causes an abnormally high conical skull shape, known as oxycephaly (also known as turricephaly or high-head).
- Premature fusion of the coronal, lambdoid and posterior sagittal sutures results in a cloverleaf skull, also known as kleeblattschädel, the most common sonographically diagnosed craniosynostosis reported in the literature because of its abnormal skull shape.

Sonographic features of the kleeblattschädel skull abnormality include an enlarged trilobed skull (**Fig. 4**), hydrocephaly, and polyhydramnios. A common error in diagnosis may be due to misinterpretation of this skull anomaly as encephalocele.[21] Kleeblattschädel abnormality is usually associated with thanatophoric dysplasia, a lethal disorder of endochondral ossification, with chondrocytes that are either decreased in number, absent, or disorganized. Thanatophoric dysplasia is considered the most common skeletal dysplasia with incidence of 1/6000 to 1/17,000 births.[22–26] There is abnormal mesenchymal-like tissue in the growth plate and periosteum, which may account for the abnormal bone formation. A far less common genetic syndrome associated with the kleeblattschädel abnormality is type II Pfeiffer syndrome, which in addition includes severe ocular proptosis, severe central nervous system involvement, and broad thumbs and great toes.

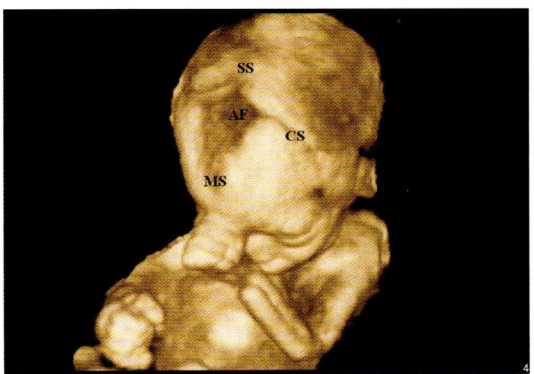

Fig. 3. Sutures and fontanelles, as imaged by 3D ultrasound reconstruction. Note the metopic, coronal, and sagittal sutures and anterior fontanelle AF, anterior fontanelle; CS, coronal suture; LS, lambdoidal suture; MS, metopic suture; PF, posterior fontanelle; SS, sagittal suture.

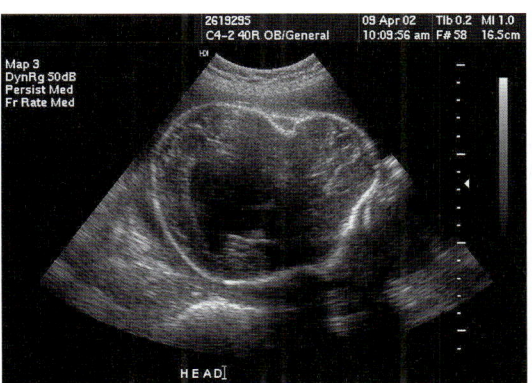

Fig. 4. Cloverleaf skull, kleeblattschädel malformation. Irregular shape of the skull, secondary to synostosis of multiple sutures. Hydrocephaly is also present. The fetus had thanatophoric dysplasia, type II.

Craniosynostosis occurs in isolation in 85% of cases but is in general described in association with several syndromes, including cranial shape abnormalities and severe malformations of the digits and grouped together under the term acrocephalosyndactyly (ACS). The Online Mendelian Inheritance in Man database contains 120 entries with craniosynostosis as an abnormal feature.[27] Five major subtypes are recognized but some overlap may exist between the various types, which makes a definite diagnosis difficult without documentation of the specific gene mutation involved.

- ACS type I, also known as Apert syndrome, is the most severe form. Findings include bicoronal facial craniosynostosis, hypertelorism, exophthalmos, midface hypoplasia, a narrow palate, and osseous or membranous syndactyly of all four extremities. There is often complete fusion of bones within the second to the fourth fingers and the presence of a single common nail, resulting in the appearance of "mitten" hands and feet. Mutations in the fibroblast growth factor 2 gene (FGFR2), which maps to chromosome 10q25-10q26, cause Apert syndrome.
- ACS type II, Crouzon syndrome, with coronal suture synostosis and facial hypoplasia. Mutations in the fibroblast growth factor 2 gene (FGFR2), which maps to chromosome 10q25-10q26, are responsible for about 90% of Crouzon syndrome, whereas about 10% of mutations in the fibroblast growth factor 3 gene (FGFR3) result in Crouzon syndrome with acanthosis nigrans. Another ACS type II form featuring sagittal, coronal, and lambdoid sutures synostosis is called Carpenter syndrome with preaxial polydactyly. Mutations in the RAB 23 gene, which is a RAS oncogene, cause this syndrome.
- ACS type III, Saethre-Chotzen syndrome with ptosis of eyelids and ears and syndactyly of second and third fingers. Mutations in the TWIST gene, which maps to chromosome 7p21-7p22, are responsible for this syndrome. Sakati-Nyhan syndrome is a variant with polysyndactyly. Advanced parental age supported new dominant mutation as the cause. No specific gene has yet been found. The Baller-Gerold syndrome shares phenotypic overlap with ACS type III but includes radial defects and is thus considered by some to be a variant. Baller-Gerold syndrome is caused by mutations in the RECQL4 gene and maps to chromosome 8q24.3.
- ACS type IV, Goodman syndrome with cleft palate, heart defects, and hermaphroditism. Goodman syndrome is believed to be a variant of Carpenter syndrome (acrocephalopolysyndactyly type II).
- ACS type V, Pfeiffer syndrome with brachycephaly, syndactyly of fingers and toes, and enlargement of the thumbs and big toes. Mutations in fibroblast growth factor 1 gene (FGFR1), which maps to chromosome 8p11.22-p12, cause Pfeiffer syndrome type I, whereas mutations in the fibroblast growth factor 2 gene (FGFR2), which maps to chromosome 10q25-10q26, cause Pfeiffer syndrome type II. Abnormalities in the hands and feet tend to be less severe in Pfeiffer syndrome type I.

Other syndromes with craniosynostosis include Shprintzen-Goldberg with craniosynostosis, with severe exophthalmos, maxillary and mandibularly hypoplasia, arachnodactyly, abdominal hernias, and developmental and mental delays resulting from mutations in the FBN1 gene (the same gene responsible for Marfan syndrome). Jackson-Weiss syndrome with midfacial hypoplasia and foot anomalies (possibly a variant of Pfeiffer) is caused by mutations in the fibroblast growth factor 2 gene (FGFR2), which maps to chromosome 10q25-10q26. Antley-Bixler syndrome is caused by mutation in the fibroblast growth factor receptor gene FGFR2 with trapezoidocephaly, midface hypoplasia, humeroradial synostosis, bowing of femora, fractures, and other abnormalities. Opitz-C (also known as Opitz trigonocephaly) syndrome results from an autosomal recessive disorder caused by an as-yet unknown gene, with microcephaly, peculiar facies, strabismus, short limbs, heart defects, and cryptorchism. There are also lesser known, multiple case reports of single patients who had craniosynostosis and a unique additional findings, named after the individual who published the case.

The diagnosis of craniosynostosis is mostly made secondary to observing other anatomic abnormalities.[12] Turribrachycephaly was identified using ultrasound study at 16 to 17 weeks in a child who had Apert syndrome, whose mother was similarly affected.[28] In these cases, typical facies may be a telltale sign (**Fig. 5**). Unilateral coronal suture synostosis, which appeared as an asymmetric multilobulated skull at 31.8 weeks' gestation, was also reported.[29] Sagittal suture craniosynostosis (scaphocephaly) was also diagnosed prenatally using ultrasound.[30–32]

Ultrasound of the Fetal Cranium

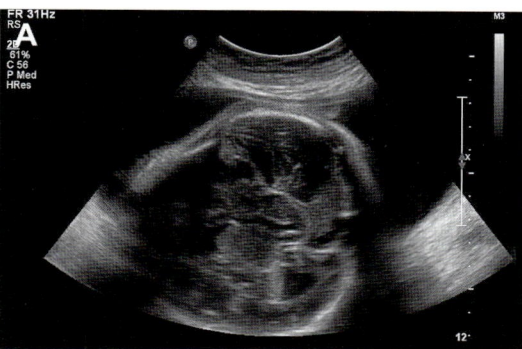 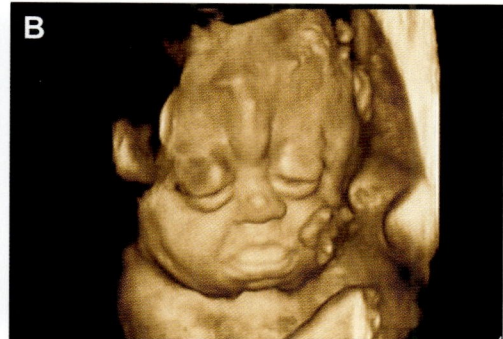

Fig. 5. Craniosynostosis. (*A*) Note the unusual skull shape, secondary to abnormal closure of sutures. (*B*) Abnormal facies, with high, prominent forehead, down-slanting eyes, exophthalmos, and bulging tongue. In addition the fetus also has low-set ears (not visible in picture). These are typical findings of Apert syndrome.

Miller and colleagues[12] examined prenatal ultrasound images of patients who had craniosynostosis to determine the extent to which prenatal diagnosis is possible. Prenatal ultrasound images of 19 patients who underwent 26 ultrasound examinations, with postnatally diagnosed metopic or coronal suture craniosynostosis, were reviewed. Diagnosis was not possible in the first trimester. All aspects of pregnancy seemed normal. In the second trimester, kleeblattschädel skull abnormality was diagnosed at 20.5 weeks, when a multilobular shape of the skull and diastasis of the frontotemporal suture was identified. In another child who had kleeblattschädel skull abnormality, the cephalic index was above normal at 86.4 and the head circumference to abdominal circumference ratio was increased. Brachycephaly was diagnosed during the second trimester. During the third trimester, the head shape deformation was more obvious.[12] The diagnosis of craniosynostosis using ultrasound may be challenging. Only 15 of 26 (58%) cases were correctly diagnosed.[12] In the same study the diagnosis of craniosynostosis was not possible during the first trimester. Diagnosis of malformations, such as kleeblattschädel, trigonocephaly, brachycephaly (bilateral coronal suture craniosynostosis), and plagiocephaly (unilateral coronal suture craniosynostosis), is possible during the second and third trimesters. Generally, craniosynostosis has an incidence rate of 52 per 100,000.[33]

An additional abnormal skull shape is described as strawberry-shaped (**Fig. 6**). This abnormal skull shape results from flattening of the occiput with pointing of the frontal bones.[34] This abnormality is commonly associated with other fetal malformations, trisomy 18, and triploidy. The ultrasonographic finding of a strawberry-shaped skull should therefore initiate a diligent search for the presence of additional markers of trisomy 18 and is a strong indication for fetal chromosome study.[34]

Abnormal Skull Findings in Neural Tube Defects

Neural tube defects (NTD) are a group of malformations resulting from incomplete closure of the neural tube by the sixth week of gestation. Such malformations are generally associated with cranial abnormalities.

Spina bifida

Spina bifida is an opening of the vertebra through which a meningeal sac may herniate out. Meningocele is defined as the meningeal sac alone; once neural elements are included in the sac the finding is referred to as meningomyelocele. Classically, fetuses who have spina bifida have one or more of the following cranial signs: small BPD, ventriculomegaly, frontal bossing ("lemon sign," ie, frontal bone scalloping),[35] elongation and downward displacement of the cerebellum ("banana sign," ie, the cerebellum is impacted deep into the posterior fossa),[36,37] and effacement or obliteration of the cisterna magna (**Fig. 7**). Examination of the fetal

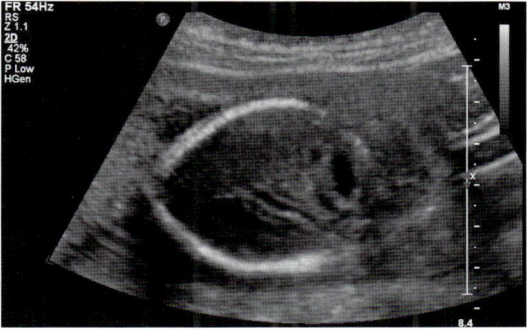

Fig. 6. Strawberry-shaped skull in a case of trisomy 18.

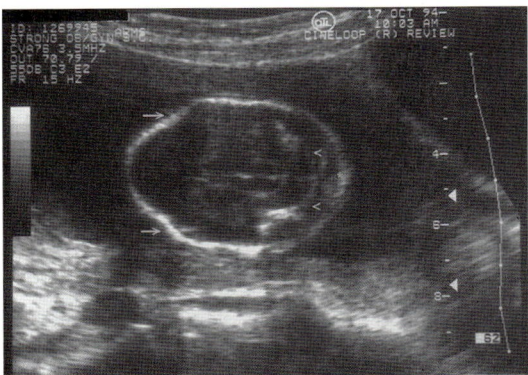

Fig. 7. Cranial signs in open spina bifida. Note in-caving of the frontal bones, resulting in the lemon shape (*arrows*), the abnormal shape of the cerebellum or banana sign (*arrowheads*) and obliteration of the posterior fossa (*asterisk*).

cranium and its contents can thus assist the in the diagnosis of open spina bifida. The sensitivity of abnormal cranial findings in correctly diagnosing spina bifida is about 99%.[37,38] The lemon sign, however, might also be present in 1% or 2% of normal fetuses. Although in most cases of spina bifida the malformation is isolated, the abnormality might be associated with chromosomal abnormalities.[39]

The incidence and diagnostic accuracy of the lemon skull deformity and the abnormal cerebellar ultrasonographic findings, as well as head size and ventriculomegaly, were evaluated in a study of 1561 patients at high risk for fetal neural tube defects.[40] In the 130 fetuses who had confirmed open spina bifida there was a gestational age–related correlation between gestational age and the presence of each of these abnormal findings. The lemon sign was present in 98% of fetuses at less than or equal to 24 weeks' gestation but in only 13% of the same fetuses at greater than 24 weeks' gestation. Cerebellar abnormalities were present in 95% of fetuses irrespective of gestational age; however, the cerebellar abnormality at less than or equal to 24 weeks' gestation was predominantly the banana sign (72%), whereas at gestations greater than 24 weeks it was cerebellar "absence" (81%). Growth restriction and cerebral ventriculomegaly significantly worsened with gestation, whereas the head circumference remained disproportionately small throughout gestation.[40]

Cephalocele

Cephalocele is defined as herniation of meninges with brain tissue through a bony defect in the skull. In most cases the lesion arises from the midline, in the occipital area, and less frequently from the parietal or frontal bones. Commonly associated conditions are either hydrocephalus due to impaired cerebrospinal fluid circulation, or microcephaly, as is the situation in massive encephalocele, when brain tissue is present inside the sac. Fetal cephalocele should be suspected whenever a para-cranial mass is seen using ultrasound. It is also commonly associated with ventriculomegaly. Because cephalocele is often associated with other malformations, detailed ultrasound examination is warranted. Proper diagnosis is possible when demonstrating the bony defect of the skull (**Fig. 8**). Nevertheless, the defect might be extremely small and impossible to demonstrate.

Neonatal mortality rate is about 40%, and mental retardation and other neurologic impairments are common among these cases.[41–45] The prenatal diagnosis of cephalocele was reported among 15 fetuses who had this skull defect. In 13 fetuses the defect was occipital, and in 1 case each with

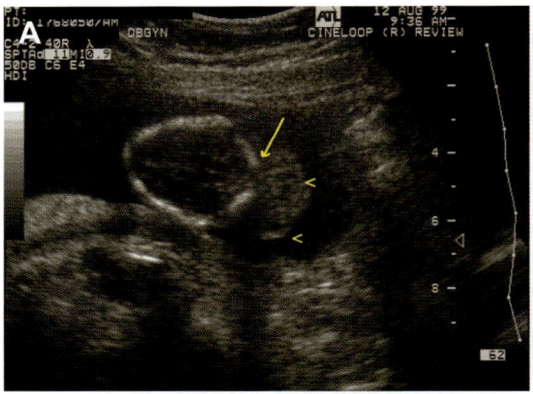
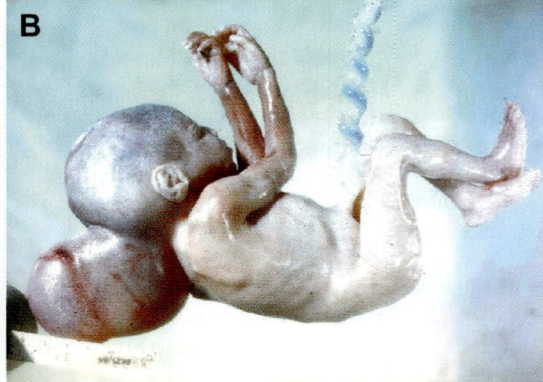

Fig. 8. Encephalocele. (*A*) Sonographic image. Note opening in occipital region (*arrow*) with extrusion of cerebral content (*arrowheads*). (*B*) Fetus after termination of pregnancy.

ethmoidal frontoparietal cephaloceles.[42] The prognosis for these fetuses was generally poor. Only 21% (3/14) were born alive, and all were handicapped. Abnormal chromosome study was noted in 44% (4/9). Associated cranial abnormalities observed in various numbers of fetuses included ventriculomegaly, the lemon sign, a flat basioccipital, "beaked" tectum, and bony defect. Likewise, in another series of 15 fetuses diagnosed with cephalocele, 11 were located in the occipital region and 2 each at the vertex and the frontonasal region.[43] Eleven fetuses were diagnosed before 24 weeks' gestation. Nine families opted for an interruption. Of the 2 pregnancies that continued to term, 1 had a benign meningocele and the other died in the neonatal period of associated cardiac anomalies. Of the 4 fetuses diagnosed after 24 weeks, 1 was normal (after surgery) at 9 months, 2 were severely handicapped, and 1 died in the immediate postpartum period.

Two genetic syndromes are important to mention in any discussion related to cephalocele: Meckel-Gruber syndrome (MKS) and Walker-Warburg syndrome. MKS is a lethal, rare, autosomal recessive condition mapped to chromosomes 17q21-24, 11q13, and 8q24. This mapping suggests genetic heterogeneity in MKS. The triad of occipital encephalocele, large polycystic kidneys, and postaxial polydactyly characterizes MKS. Associated abnormalities include oral clefting, genital anomalies, CNS malformations, and liver fibrosis. Pulmonary hypoplasia is the leading cause of death. Improvements in ultrasonography have enabled prenatal diagnosis as early as 10 weeks' gestation. The clinical features of Walker-Warburg syndrome are congenital cataracts, microphthalmia, occipital encephalocele, fusion of the hemispheres, and absence of the corpus callosum. Mutations in two genes, *POMT1* and *POMT2*, were found in some but not all affected cases. Additional genes coding for glycosyltransferases, yet to be identified, are believed to be the major cause of this disorder.

Anencephaly

Anencephaly is a lethal defect characterized by absence of the brain and cranium above the base of the skull. It is considered by some as the final stage of acrania (aka, exencephaly).[46] In acrania, the upper part of the calvaria is absent with abnormal brain substance visible (**Fig. 9**). It is believed to occur during the beginning of week four of the pregnancy. At that time the anterior neuropore is expected to close. The membrane that is normally destined to become the epidermis remains membranous and normal migration of mesenchymal tissue does not occur. The result is normal base but absent calvarial bones of the skull and dura mater. The brain tissue that is now unprotected by the calvaria is disrupted, resulting in anencephaly.[47–50] In anencephaly, no anatomic structure is visible above the forehead line (**Fig. 10**). Amniotic bands may occasionally be an important etiologic factor.[51] Associated malformations are extremely common with anencephaly and include spina bifida, cleft lip and palate, club foot, omphalocele, and hydramnion. Acrania and anencephaly can be reliably diagnosed at the routine 10- to 14-week ultrasound scan, provided study includes demonstration of a normal-appearing fetal brain and skull.[52] Before 10 weeks of gestation, diagnosis may be difficult because of lack of adequate calcification of the calvaria.

MICROCEPHALY

Microcephaly (ie, severely small head) is defined as head circumference at least 3 SDs below the mean.[53–56] It is primarily a brain development disorder with secondary deficient growth of the skull.

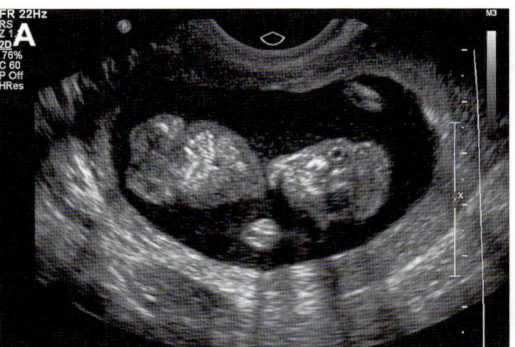 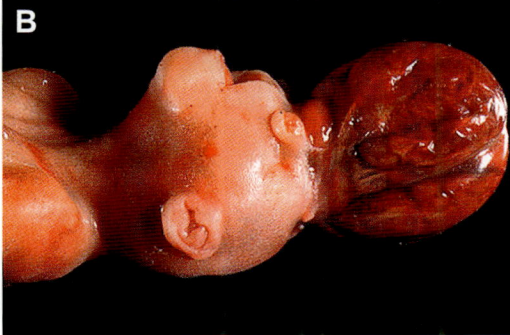

Fig. 9. (*A, B*) Acrania (exencephaly), 2D and 3D images and gross pathology. Note the absence of upper the cranium and amorphous brain material above the orbits.

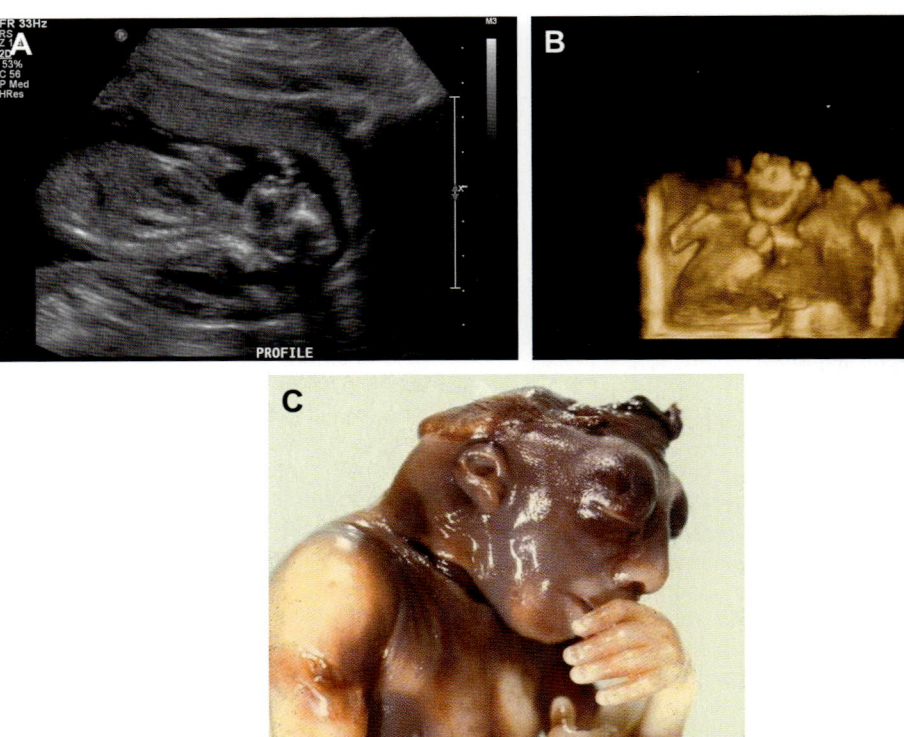

Fig. 10. Anencephaly. Note absence of cranium and contents above the eye-line. Compare with **Fig. 9.** (*A*) 2D image of the fetal head. (*B*) 3D reconstructed image. (*C*) The fetus following termination of pregnancy.

This condition is commonly associated with environmental insults (alcohol, radiation, toluene abuse, anorexia, infections) or genetic disorders (trisomies 18 and 13 and other chromosome abnormality and genetic syndromes).[53,56,57] Tolmie and colleagues[56] described a series of 29 isolated cases of microcephaly and 9 families with recurrent microcephaly. The recurrence risk for sibs was 19%, which reflects the high incidence of autosomal recessive disorders associated with microcephaly in this study and in other studies. Anatomic shortening of the fetal frontal lobe seems to precede microcephaly.[53] Brain size determines the size of the calvaria.[58] Biometry of the frontal lobe of the fetal brain may be a valuable tool for the identification of the fetus at risk for microcephaly.[53] Careful study of the of the developing fetal brain is necessary in suspicious cases, because abnormalities of neurocranial architecture occur in approximately two thirds of cases.[53]

MR imaging can add significant information to the ultrasound examination.[59] Steinlin and colleagues[59] found MR imaging revealed significant abnormalities in the majority of infants who had primary microcephaly and neurodevelopmental delays, and seems to be more sensitive than cranial ultrasound and CT. Interestingly, the underlying conditions that may predispose to brain atrophy may be recognizable using Doppler ultrasonography, suggesting the usefulness of brain vasculature imaging.[60]

THE ABNORMAL SKULL IN OTHER GENETIC DISORDERS
Osteogenesis Imperfecta

Osteogenesis imperfecta (OI) is a heterogeneous genetic disorder with defective type 1 collagen attributable to mutations in two type 1 collagen genes, COL1A1 and COL1A2. The disorder is characterized by osteopenia, bone fractures, and blue sclera.[61,62] Nonlethal forms are associated with impaired hearing, poor dentition, and hypermobile joints. Ultrasound examination demonstrates variable hypomineralization and in utero bone fractures in some but not all forms of OI.[63] Hypomineralization of the skull may be severe, resulting in complete absence of posterior acoustic shadowing, leading to easy sonographic demonstration of the ventricles and choroids plexus. Additional findings may include micromelia, irregularity and bowing of bones, and bell-shaped thorax. A peculiar finding is indentation of the fetal skull secondary to the hypomineralization and caused by transducer pressure (**Fig. 11**). The differential diagnosis should include other micromelic dysplasias and conditions leading to hypomineralization of the bones, such as hypophosphatasia or achondrogenesis.

Congenital Hypophosphatasia

Although formal diagnostic criteria are not established, all forms of hypophosphatasia (except pseudo-hypophosphatasia) share in common reduced activity of unfractionated serum alkaline phosphatase (ALP) and presence of either one or two pathologic mutations in *ALPL*, the gene encoding alkaline phosphatase, tissue-nonspecific isozyme (TNSALP). Perinatal and infantile hypophosphatasia are inherited in an autosomal recessive manner. The milder forms, especially adult and odontohypophosphatasia, may be inherited in an autosomal recessive or autosomal dominant manner depending on the *ALPL* mutation effect on TNSALP. Because of deficiency in alkaline phosphatase activity, the phenotypic abnormalities result from impaired ossification.[64–66] Ultrasound might demonstrate profound under-ossification of bones, a hypoechogenic skull, bowing and shortening of long bones, and severe micromelia.[64–66] Severe under-ossification of the skull may result in a membranous skull, which is compressible and may be mistaken for acrania.[67]

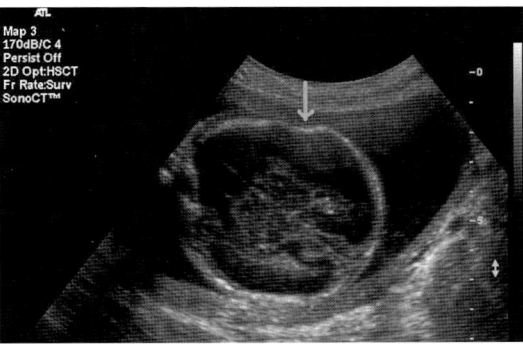

Fig. 11. A case of perinatal lethal (type II) osteogenesis imperfecta. Note depression of proximal skull (*arrow*) secondary to transducer pressure.

Radiologic examination can occasionally help in the diagnosis of the under-ossification.[67]

Abnormal Ossification

Abnormal skull ossification can be attributed to various drugs, and specifically angiotensin-converting enzyme (ACE) inhibitors and folic acid antagonists.[68,69] ACE inhibitors are widely used for controlling hypertension.[70] Their use in pregnant women increases the risk for fetotoxicity.[71] ACE inhibitor fetopathy is characterized by hypoplastic skull bones (hypocalvaria),[70,71] in addition to fetal hypotension, oligohydramnios, growth restriction, pulmonary hypoplasia, and renal tubular dysplasia. Although the true frequency of adverse fetal effects is unclear, because of the debilitating and lethal nature of the fetal damage it is highly recommended to avoid exposure to ACE inhibitors during pregnancy, particularly during the second and third trimesters.

THREE-DIMENSIONAL ULTRASOUND OF THE FETAL CRANIUM

Three-dimensional ultrasound technology can be a useful adjunct to two-dimensional (2D) examination and for parental counseling.[72–78] The stereoscopic display of rendered 3D ultrasound data adds valuable information that assists in identification of fetal bony structures, such as cranial sutures, particularly in complex formations. The increasing availability of stereoscopic visualization workstations will offer an additional tool for fetal diagnosis and evaluation.[3]

Roelfsema and colleagues[79] explored the development of the fetal skull base using 3D sonography. The researchers performed serial 3D sonographic measurements of the anterior skull base length, posterior cranial fossa length, and skull base angle in 126 normal singleton pregnancies at 18 to 34 weeks of gestation. Measurements were technically successful in 69% to 94% of cases. A statistically significant gestational age-related increase was established for both the anterior skull base length and the posterior cranial fossa length. The skull base angle showed a small but significant flexion of about 6 degrees. The reproducibility was acceptable for all fetal skull base measurements.[79] Three-dimensional ultrasound was also used to describe patterns of abnormal development of the metopic suture in association with fetal malformations during the second and third trimesters of pregnancy.[75] A cross-sectional study of the frontal bones and metopic suture in 11 fetuses at 17 to 32 weeks of gestation was performed. Cases were selected because obvious abnormalities in the metopic

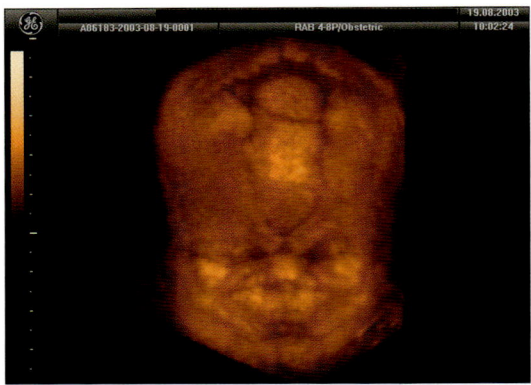

Fig. 12. Abnormal metopic suture. In addition, the fetus was found to have club feet, cerebellar hypoplasia, intracranial cyst, and agenesis of the corpus callosum. (*Courtesy of* Dr. Bernard Benoit, Nice, France.)

sutures were noted. In each case, the malformation was initially detected by 2D ultrasound study and subsequently 3D ultrasound technology using transparent maximum imaging mode was applied. Four patterns of abnormality in the metopic suture were identified:

- Delayed development with a V- or Y-shaped open suture, which is found in normal fetuses at 12 to 16 weeks.
- U-shaped open suture, presumably because of upward growth of the frontal bones with delayed closure.
- Premature closure of the suture, which is normally observed after 32 weeks.
- The presence of additional bone between the frontal bones (**Fig. 12**).[75]

Premature closure of the suture or the finding of additional bone between the frontal bones was observed in fetuses who had holoprosencephaly and abnormalities of the corpus callosum, whereas the V-, Y-, and U-shaped metopic sutures were observed in fetuses who had facial defects involving the orbits, nasal bones, lip, palate, and mandible, in the absence of holoprosencephaly and abnormal corpus callosum.[75]

SUMMARY

Fetal cranial defects and abnormal skull shape are amenable to ultrasound study diagnosis. Correct identification of the nature of the abnormality is extremely important and helpful in establishing diagnosis and long-term prognosis. In addition it might direct the care provider to apply the correct genetic study, chromosome or DNA related, for final diagnosis confirmation. The astute operator is likely to immediately suspect a problem in the face of fetal microcephaly, ossification abnormality, bone fractures, and abnormal skull shape secondary to craniosynostosis or brain structure abnormality. Although most of these abnormalities are amenable to 2D ultrasound study detection, 3D ultrasound and infrequently fetal MR imaging can be an adjunct for delineation of cranial abnormalities and may be useful in demonstrating the extent of the abnormality and in parental counseling.

REFERENCES

1. Crelin ES. Development of the musculoskeletal system. Clin Symp 1981;33(1):1–36.
2. Zorzoli A, Kustermann A, Caravelli E, et al. Measurements of fetal limb bones in early pregnancy. Ultrasound Obstet Gynecol 1994;4(1):29–33.
3. Nelson TR, Ji EK, Lee JH, et al. Stereoscopic evaluation of fetal bony structures. J Ultrasound Med 2008;27(1):15–24.
4. Pretorius DH, Nelson TR. Prenatal visualization of cranial sutures and fontanelles with three-dimensional ultrasonography. J Ultrasound Med 1994;13(11):871–6.
5. Willocks J, Donald I, Duggan TC, et al. Foetal cephalometry by ultrasound. J Obstet Gynaecol Br Commonw 1964;71:11–20.
6. Jeanty P, Cantraine F, Cousaert E, et al. The binocular distance: a new way to estimate fetal age. J Ultrasound Med 1984;3(6):241–3.
7. Borenstein M, Dagklis T, Csapo B, et al. Brachycephaly and frontal lobe hypoplasia in fetuses with trisomy 21 at 11 + 0 to 13 + 6 weeks. Ultrasound Obstet Gynecol 2006;28(7):870–5.
8. Levine D, Kilpatrick S, Damato N, et al. Dolichocephaly and oligohydramnios in preterm premature rupture of the membranes. J Ultrasound Med 1996;15(5):375–9.
9. Hadlock FP, Deter RL, Carpenter RJ, et al. Estimating fetal age: effect of head shape on BPD. AJR Am J Roentgenol 1981;137(1):83–5.
10. Houlton MC, Brennan DT. Dolichocephaly—a source of error in serial cephalometry. Br J Obstet Gynaecol 1976;83(4):276–8.
11. Borrell A, Costa D, Martinez JM, et al. Brachycephaly is ineffective for detection of Down syndrome in early midtrimester fetuses. Early Hum Dev 1997;47(1):57–61.
12. Miller C, Losken HW, Towbin R, et al. Ultrasound diagnosis of craniosynostosis. Cleft Palate Craniofac J 2002;39(1):73–80.
13. Sukcharoen N, Tannirandorn Y, Suwajanakorn S, et al. Biparietal diameter/femur length ratio and actual femur length/expected femur length ratio: a sonographic

screening method for Down's syndrome. J Med Assoc Thai 1992;75(8):483–7.
14. Tran LT, Carr DB, Mitsumori LM, et al. Second-trimester biparietal diameter/nasal bone length ratio is an independent predictor of trisomy 21. J Ultrasound Med 2005;24(6):805–10.
15. Witt PD, Hardesty RA, Zuppan C, et al. Fetal kleeblattschädel cranium: morphologic, radiographic, and histologic analysis. Cleft Palate Craniofac J 1992;29(4):363–8.
16. Jeanty P, Romero R, Staudach A, et al. Facial anatomy of the fetus. J Ultrasound Med 1986;5(11): 607–16.
17. Brahman S, Jenna R, Wittenauer HJ. Sonographic in utero appearance of Kleeblattschädel syndrome. J Clin Ultrasound 1979;7(6):481–4.
18. Burrows PE, Stannard MW, Pearrow J, et al. Early antenatal sonographic recognition of thanatophoric dysplasia with cloverleaf skull deformity. AJR Am J Roentgenol 1984;143(4):841–3.
19. Cohen MM Jr. Craniosynostosis update 1987. Am J Med Genet Suppl 1988;4:99–148.
20. Kabbani H, Raghuveer TS. Craniosynostosis. Am Fam Physician 2004;69(12):2863–70.
21. Stamm ER, Pretorius DH, Rumack CM, et al. Kleeblattschädel anomaly. In utero sonographic appearance. J Ultrasound Med 1987;6(6): 319–24.
22. Fasanelli S, Kozlowski K, Reiter S, et al. Dyssegmental dysplasia (report of two cases with a review of the literature). Skeletal Radiol 1985;14(3):173–7.
23. Indu PS, Poothiode U, Augustine J, et al. Thanatophoric dysplasia: a case report and review of literature. Indian J Pathol Microbiol 2007;50(3):589–92.
24. Kozlowski K, Warren PS, Fisher CC. Cloverleaf skull with generalised bone dysplasia. Report of a case with short review of the literature. Pediatr Radiol 1985;15(6):412–4.
25. Kremens B, Kemperdick H, Borchard F, et al. Thanatophoric dysplasia with cloverleaf-skull. Case report and review of the literature. Eur J Pediatr 1982; 139(4):298–303.
26. Schild RL, Hunt GH, Moore J, et al. Antenatal sonographic diagnosis of thanatophoric dysplasia: a report of three cases and a review of the literature with special emphasis on the differential diagnosis. Ultrasound Obstet Gynecol 1996;8(1):62–7.
27. McKusick VA. OMIM, Online Mendelian Inheritance in Man. Available at: http://www.ncbi.nlm.nih.gov/omim/. Accessed February 14, 2008.
28. Narayan H, Scott IV. Prenatal ultrasound diagnosis of Apert's syndrome. Prenat Diagn 1991;11(3): 187–92.
29. Meilstrup JW, Botti JJ, MacKay DR, et al. Prenatal sonographic appearance of asymmetric craniosynostosis: a case report. J Ultrasound Med 1995; 14(4):307–10.
30. Huang HW, Lin H, Chang SY, et al. Isolated craniosynostosis: prenatal ultrasound of scaphocephaly with polyhydramnios. Chang Gung Med J 2001;24(12): 816–9.
31. Pooh RK, Nakagawa Y, Nagamachi N, et al. Transvaginal sonography of the fetal brain: detection of abnormal morphology and circulation. Croat Med J 1998;39(2):147–57.
32. van der Ham LI, Cohen-Overbeek TE, Paz y Geuze HD, et al. The ultrasonic detection of an isolated craniosynostosis. Prenat Diagn 1995;15(12): 1189–92.
33. Hegge FN, Franklin RW, Watson PT, et al. Fetal malformations commonly detectable on obstetric ultrasound. J Reprod Med 1990;35(4):391–8.
34. Nicolaides KH, Salvesen DR, Snijders RJ, et al. Strawberry-shaped skull in fetal trisomy 18. Fetal Diagn Ther 1992;7(2):132–7.
35. Filly RA. The "lemon" sign: a clinical perspective. Radiology 1988;167(2):573–5.
36. Johnson DD, Nager CW, Budorick NE. False-positive diagnosis of spina bifida in a fetus with triploidy. Obstet Gynecol 1997;89(5 Pt 2):809–11.
37. Blumenfeld Z, Siegler E, Bronshtein M. The early diagnosis of neural tube defects. Prenat Diagn 1993; 13(9):863–71.
38. Watson WJ, Chescheir NC, Katz VL, et al. The role of ultrasound in evaluation of patients with elevated maternal serum alpha-fetoprotein: a review. Obstet Gynecol 1991;78(1):123–8.
39. Babcook CJ, Goldstein RB, Filly RA. Prenatally detected fetal myelomeningocele: is karyotype analysis warranted? Radiology 1995;194(2):491–4.
40. Van den Hof MC, Nicolaides KH, Campbell J, et al. Evaluation of the lemon and banana signs in one hundred thirty fetuses with open spina bifida. Am J Obstet Gynecol 1990;162(2):322–7.
41. Budorick NE, Pretorius DH, McGahan JP, et al. Cephalocele detection in utero: sonographic and clinical features. Ultrasound Obstet Gynecol 1995; 5(2):77–85.
42. Goldstein RB, LaPidus AS, Filly RA. Fetal cephaloceles: diagnosis with US. Radiology 1991;180(3): 803–8.
43. Jeanty P, Shah D, Zaleski W, et al. Prenatal diagnosis of fetal cephalocele: a sonographic spectrum. Am J Perinatol 1991;8(2):144–9.
44. Nicolini U, Ferrazzi E, Kustermann A, et al. Effectiveness of routine ultrasound in screening congenital defects. J Perinat Med 1982;10(2):125–9.
45. Wininger SJ, Donnenfeld AE. Syndromes identified in fetuses with prenatally diagnosed cephaloceles. Prenat Diagn 1994;14(9):839–43.
46. Cafici D, Sepulveda W. First-trimester echogenic amniotic fluid in the acrania-anencephaly sequence. J Ultrasound Med 2003;22(10):1075–9 [quiz 1080–1].

47. Hautman GD, Sherman SJ, Utter GO, et al. Acrania. J Ultrasound Med 1995;14(7):552–4.
48. Doray B, Favre R, Gasser B, et al. Recurrent neural tube defects associated with partial trisomy 2p22-pter: report of two siblings and review of the literature. Genet Couns 2003;14(2):165–72.
49. Koukoura O, Sifakis S, Stratoudakis G, et al. A case report of recurrent anencephaly and literature review. Clin Exp Obstet Gynecol 2006;33(3):185–9.
50. Timor-Tritsch IE, Greenebaum E, Monteagudo A, et al. Exencephaly-anencephaly sequence: proof by ultrasound imaging and amniotic fluid cytology. J Matern Fetal Med 1996;5(4):182–5.
51. Cincore V, Ninios AP, Pavlik J, et al. Prenatal diagnosis of acrania associated with amniotic band syndrome. Obstet Gynecol 2003;102(5 Pt 2):1176–8.
52. Johnson SP, Sebire NJ, Snijders RJ, et al. Ultrasound screening for anencephaly at 10-14 weeks of gestation. Ultrasound Obstet Gynecol 1997;9(1):14–6.
53. Persutte WH. Microcephaly—no small deal. Ultrasound Obstet Gynecol 1998;11(5):317–8.
54. Gabis L, Gelman-Kohan Z, Mogilner M. Microcephaly due to fetal brain disruption sequence. Case report. J Perinat Med 1997;25(2):213–5.
55. Majoor-Krakauer DF, Wladimiroff JW, Stewart PA, et al. Microcephaly, micrognathia, and bird-headed dwarfism: prenatal diagnosis of a Seckel-like syndrome. Am J Med Genet 1987;27(1):183–8.
56. Tolmie JL, McNay M, Stephenson JB, et al. Microcephaly: genetic counseling and antenatal diagnosis after the birth of an affected child. Am J Med Genet 1987;27(3):583–94.
57. Chow G, Padfield CJ. A case of infantile neuroaxonal dystrophy-connatal seitelberger disease. J Child Neurol 2008;23:418–20.
58. Pilu G, Rizzo N, Orsini LF, et al. Antenatal recognition of cerebral anomalies. Ultrasound Med Biol 1986;12(4):319–26.
59. Steinlin M, Zurrer M, Martin E, et al. Contribution of magnetic resonance imaging in the evaluation of microcephaly. Neuropediatrics 1991;22(4):184–9.
60. Pilu G, Falco P, Milano V, et al. Prenatal diagnosis of microcephaly assisted by vaginal sonography and power Doppler. Ultrasound Obstet Gynecol 1998;11(5):357–60.
61. Huang RP, Ambrose CG, Sullivan E, et al. Functional significance of bone density measurements in children with osteogenesis imperfecta. J Bone Joint Surg Am 2006;88(6):1324–30.
62. Martin E, Shapiro JR. Osteogenesis imperfecta: epidemiology and pathophysiology. Curr Osteoporos Rep 2007;5(3):91–7.
63. Tongsong T, Wanapirak C, Siriangkul S. Prenatal diagnosis of osteogenesis imperfecta type II. Int J Gynaecol Obstet 1998;61(1):33–8.
64. Gortzak-Uzan L, Sheiner E, Gohar J. Prenatal diagnosis of congenital hypophosphatasia in a consanguineous Bedouin couple. A case report. J Reprod Med 2000;45(7):588–90.
65. Tongsong T, Pongsatha S. Early prenatal sonographic diagnosis of congenital hypophosphatasia. Ultrasound Obstet Gynecol 2000;15(3):252–5.
66. Tongsong T, Sirichotiyakul S, Siriangkul S. Prenatal diagnosis of congenital hypophosohatasia. J Clin Ultrasound 1995;23(1):52–5.
67. DeLange M, Rouse GA. Prenatal diagnosis of hypophosphatasia. J Ultrasound Med 1990;9(2):115–7.
68. Torikai E, Kageyama Y, Takahashi M, et al. The effect of methotrexate on bone metabolism markers in patients with rheumatoid arthritis. Mod Rheumatol 2006;16(6):350–4.
69. Barr M Jr, Cohen MM Jr. ACE inhibitor fetopathy and hypocalvaria: the kidney-skull connection. Teratology 1991;44(5):485–95.
70. Pryde PG, Sedman AB, Nugent CE, et al. Angiotensin-converting enzyme inhibitor fetopathy. J Am Soc Nephrol 1993;3(9):1575–82.
71. Schaefer C. Angiotensin II-receptor-antagonists: further evidence of fetotoxicity but not teratogenicity. Birth Defects Res A Clin Mol Teratol 2003;67(8):591–4.
72. David AL, Turnbull C, Scott R, et al. Diagnosis of Apert syndrome in the second-trimester using 2D and 3D ultrasound. Prenat Diagn 2007;27(7):629–32.
73. Benacerraf BR, Spiro R, Mitchell AG. Using three-dimensional ultrasound to detect craniosynostosis in a fetus with Pfeiffer syndrome. Ultrasound Obstet Gynecol 2000;16(4):391–4.
74. Benoit B, Chaoui R. Three-dimensional ultrasound with maximal mode rendering: a novel technique for the diagnosis of bilateral or unilateral absence or hypoplasia of nasal bones in second-trimester screening for Down syndrome. Ultrasound Obstet Gynecol 2005;25(1):19–24.
75. Chaoui R, Levaillant JM, Benoit B, et al. Three-dimensional sonographic description of abnormal metopic suture in second- and third-trimester fetuses. Ultrasound Obstet Gynecol 2005;26(7):761–4.
76. Dagklis T, Borenstein M, Peralta CF, et al. Three-dimensional evaluation of mid-facial hypoplasia in fetuses with trisomy 21 at 11 + 0 to 13 + 6 weeks of gestation. Ultrasound Obstet Gynecol 2006;28(3):261–5.
77. Roelfsema NM, Hop WC, Wladimiroff JW. Three-dimensional sonographic determination of normal fetal mandibular and maxillary size during the second half of pregnancy. Ultrasound Obstet Gynecol 2006;28(7):950–7.
78. Lee A, Deutinger J, Bernaschek G. Three dimensional ultrasound: abnormalities of the fetal face in surface and volume rendering mode. Br J Obstet Gynaecol 1995;102(4):302–6.
79. Roelfsema NM, Grijseels EW, Hop WC, et al. Three-dimensional sonography of prenatal skull base development. Ultrasound Obstet Gynecol 2007;29(4):372–7.

Diagnostic Approach to Prenatally Diagnosed Limb Abnormalities

Arie Koifman, MD[a,b,c], Ori Nevo, MD[d], Ants Toi, MD[e], David Chitayat, MD[a,b,c],*

KEYWORDS

- Detection and diagnosis of limb abnormalities using prenatal ultrasound

The prevalence of limb abnormalities is approximately six in 10,000 live births, with higher incidence in the upper limbs compared with the lower limbs (3.4 of 10,000 and 1.1 of 10,000, respectively).[1] Unilateral limb abnormalities are more common than bilateral and are more frequent in the right limb compared with the left.[2]

Limb formation occurs early in embryogenesis (4–8 weeks' gestation), whereas primary ossification centers are present in all the long bones of the limbs by the 12th week of gestation. Development of the upper and lower limbs is similar except that the morphogenesis of the lower limb lags approximately 1 to 2 days behind that of the upper limb. The molecular regulation of limb formation is complex and involves different gene families. The homeobox (HOX) gene family has a key role in the positioning of the limbs along the craniocaudal axis in the flank regions of the embryo. Limb outgrowth is tightly regulated by fibroblast growth factor (FGF) genes along with the bone morphogenetic proteins (BMPs). Patterning of the anteroposterior axis of the limb is regulated by sonic hedgehog (SHH) genes, contributing to the correct order of appearance of digits. SHH genes are under different regulatory transcription factors (BMPs, EN1, WNT7a, and others),[3,4,5] and the transcription factors TBX5 and TBX4 regulate the differentiation of upper from lower limbs.[6]

The detection and diagnosis of limb abnormalities using prenatal ultrasonography depends on patient body habitus, quality of the ultrasound machine, and operator skill and capabilities.[7] Studies have shown that limb abnormalities were diagnosed more accurately when associated with other abnormalities and when detected as part of a known syndrome (chromosomal or single gene), whereas isolated limb defects were less likely to be diagnosed prenatally.[7,8] Holder-Espinasse and colleagues,[9] in their series of 107 cases of limb abnormalities detected prenatally, concluded that diagnosis was reached in 79% of the overall cases, whereas only 29% were diagnosed as isolated limb malformations. The limb abnormality was not diagnosed in 21% of the cases. The authors concluded that familiarity with genetic syndromes is very helpful in reaching a diagnosis, particularly if the anomaly is associated with other malformations.

---

[a] The Prenatal Diagnosis and Medical Genetics Program, Mount Sinai Hospital, University of Toronto, The Ontario Power Generation Building, 700 University Avenue, Rm. 3292, Toronto, ON, Canada M5G 1X5
[b] Department of Obstetrics and Gynecology, Mount Sinai Hospital, University of Toronto, 92 College Street, Toronto, ON, Canada M5G 1L4
[c] The Hospital for Sick Children, Division of Clinical and Metabolic Genetics, University of Toronto, 555 University Avenue, Toronto, ON, Canada M5G 1X8
[d] Department of Obstetrics and Gynecology, Sunnybrook Health Sciences Centre, University of Toronto, 76 Grenville Street (at Women's College Hospital), Toronto, ON, Canada M5S 1B2
[e] Department of Diagnostic Imaging, Mount Sinai Hospital, University of Toronto, The Ontario Power Generation Building, 700 University Avenue, Rm. 3292, Toronto, ON, Canada M5G 1X5
* Corresponding author. The Prenatal Diagnosis and Medical Genetics Program, Mount Sinai Hospital, The Ontario Power Generation Building, 700 University Avenue, Rm. 3292, Toronto, Ontario, Canada, M5G 1X5.
E-mail address: dchitayat@mtsinai.on.ca (D. Chitayat).

Upper and lower limb abnormalities are a morphologically and etiologically heterogeneous group of abnormalities. They include malformation, deformation, or disruption and can be limited to one limb or part of a limb. Limb anomalies may affect only the upper or the lower limbs, or all four limbs and can be isolated or associated with other abnormalities. These defects are frequently acquired or multifactorial in origin but are occasionally inherited. Although single gene disorders,[9,10,11] chromosomal abnormalities,[5] intrauterine factors,[12] vascular events,[3,13] maternal diseases,[14] and maternal exposures[8,15] are all known causes of limb abnormalities, in many cases the etiology remains unknown.

One of the challenges in providing medical care for patients with fetal limb anomaly is to define the etiology of the disorder and thus the prognosis and recurrence risk for future pregnancies. This knowledge will provide the parents with accurate information regarding the possibilities for prenatal diagnosis for their future pregnancies and, if possible, options for prevention of recurrence. The effort to delineate the etiology of a limb defect should involve a multidisciplinary approach including the obstetrician, radiologist/sonologist, clinical geneticist, neonatologist/pediatrician, and a pediatric orthopedic surgeon. Other specialties may be needed if other abnormalities are noted.

The aim of this review is to describe the diagnostic approach to prenatally detectable limb abnormalities using detailed fetal ultrasonography.

STEPWISE APPROACH TO THE FETUS WITH PRENATALLY DIAGNOSED LIMB ABNORMALITIES—ASSEMBLING THE PUZZLE
Step I—Describe the Limb Abnormalities Using Appropriate Terms

Once a limb abnormality is identified, the first step in the clinical workup is careful description of the abnormality using established nomenclature (**Table 1**). Stoll and colleagues,[16] published a useful classification and description of limb defects in the European Surveillance of Congenital Anomalies (EUROCAT) guide. This classification scheme is based on a descriptive rather than etiologic approach, although a specific condition can fit more than one category.

The operator should strictly adhere to the below-listed definition of malformation, deformation, or disruption to correctly categorize the defect from a pathogenetic point of view because this has utmost importance in determining etiology, prognosis, and recurrence risk.

- *Malformation*: A morphologic defect at an organ, part of an organ, or larger region of the body resulting from an intrinsically abnormal developmental process (eg, ectrodactyly, phocomelia, polydactyly).
- *Deformation*: An abnormal form, shape, or position of part of the body caused by mechanical forces (eg, clubfeet, genu recurvatum).
- *Disruption*: A morphologic defect of an organ, part of an organ, or a segment of the body resulting from the extrinsic breakdown of, or an interference with, an originally normal developmental process (eg, amniotic band sequence).

Step II—Look for Other Abnormalities (Isolated versus Nonisolated Limb Abnormalities)

When limb abnormalities are associated with other detectable abnormalities they are more likely to result from chromosomal abnormalities, single gene disorders, or teratogenic exposure and are less likely the result of a multifactorial condition or vascular injury. However, because not all fetal abnormalities can be detected by fetal ultrasonography, what is thought to be an isolated limb abnormality prenatally may actually be multiple abnormalities noted postnatally. Moreover, an apparently mild single abnormality may later be established as a major disorder (eg, clubfeet that are associated with brain abnormalities or metabolic disorder). If there is a family history of a medical condition, it is important to provide this information to the sonographer, along with a list of the abnormalities associated with the condition, in an attempt to help detect subtle and uncommon but important findings. For example, the standard ultrasound examination is unlikely to detect epiphyseal calcifications. However, these are visible if specifically sought.

The sonologist should try to further define the nature of the limb abnormality by adhering to the following pattern of abnormalities:

- *Dysplasia*: An abnormal organization of cells into tissue(s) and its morphologic result(s). In other words, a process (and the consequence) of dishistiogenesis.
- *Sequence*: A pattern of multiple anomalies derived from a single known or presumed prior anomaly or mechanical factor.
- *Syndrome*: A recognized pattern of developmentally independent malformations having one etiology.
- *Association*: Nonrandom concurrence of independent malformations, the etiology of which (single or multiple) is unknown. This includes the VACTERL association: Vertebral defects, Anal atresia, Cardiac

Table 1
Nomenclature used in defining the type of limb defect

Acheiria	Absence of Hand(s)
Acromelia	Shortening of a distal segment in hands/feet
Adactyly	Absence of fingers/toes
Amelia	Absence of a limb(s)
Apodia	Absence of foot/feet
Brachydactyly	Abnormally short fingers
Camptomelia	Bent limb
Clinodactyly	Inturning of a finger
Hemimelia	Absence of a longitudinal segment of a limb
Mesomelia	Shortening of a middle segment in hands/feet
Micromelia	Shortening of all long bones
Oligodactyly	Partial loss of fingers
Phocomelia	Hypoplasia of the limbs (hands attached to shoulders, feet to hips)
Polydactyly	Supernumerary digits
Rhizomelia	Shortening of a proximal segment in upper/lower limbs (humeri/femurs)
Syndactyly	Fused digits
Terminal Transverse defects	Absence of distal structures of the limb with normal proximal structure
Proximal intercalary defects	Absence or severe hypoplasia of proximal intercalary parts of the limb where the distal parts of the limb (normal or malformed), are present
Longitudinal absence or severe hypoplasia of a lateral part of the limb	Absence of a lateral component of a limb
Split hand/foot (ectrodactyly)	Absence of central digits with or without absence of central metacarpal/metatarsal bones. Usually associated with syndactyly of other digits.
Multiple types of reduction defects	More than one defect of those listed above in the same individual

abnormalities, T-E fistula, Esophageal atresia, Renal dysplasia, and Limb/radial abnormalities.

Step III—Obtain the Pregnancy History

The pregnancy history should include information regarding maternal diseases such as diabetes mellitus, hypercoagulability, systemic lupus erythematosus and other autoimmune diseases, myotonic dystrophy, high blood pressure, and exposure to teratogens such as medications, infections, alcohol, and cigarette smoke.

Step IV—Obtain the Family History

A three-generation family history should be obtained, using standardized pedigree symbols,[15] that contains critical medical data and biological relationships. Information regarding family members with congenital limb or other abnormalities, recurrent miscarriages, stillbirths, mental retardation, inherited conditions, and consanguinity should be included. Obtaining medical records from specific family members for documentation and accurate counseling may be required. In general, a family pedigree is a tool for making a medical diagnosis, deciding on testing strategies, establishing the pattern of inheritance, identifying at-risk family members, calculating risks, determining reproductive options, distinguishing genetic from other risk factors, making decisions on medical management and surveillance, developing patient rapport, educating the patient, and exploring the patient's understanding.[1] If new and important information becomes available, it may be worthwhile repeating the ultrasound examination because it may detect abnormalities that were not specifically sought during the initial examination.

Table 2
Chromosomal disorders associated with limb abnormalities

Chromosome Abnormality	Limb Abnormalities
Trisomy 21	Short broad hands, clinodactyly and short fifth fingers, "sandal gap," slightly short femur and humerus
Trisomy 13	Postaxial polydactyly, clenched hands, overlapping fingers, prominent heels
Trisomy 18	Radial ray defects, hypoplastic thumbs, clenched hands, overlapping fingers, "rocker bottom feet," clubhand, clubfeet, ectrodactyly, prominent heels, dislocated hips
del(4) (p16.3)	Clubfeet
del(5) (p15.3)	Clinodactyly of the fifth fingers, clubfeet, syndactyly of the second and third fingers and toes, oligosyndactyly, hyperextensible joints
Trisomy 8	Camptodactyly of second to fifth fingers, joint contractures
Triploidy	Syndactyly of the third to fourth fingers, "sandal gap", clubfeet
Del(3) (p25-pter)	Postaxial polydactyly

Step V—Compile the Information and Form a Differential Diagnosis

The existence of a limb abnormality on fetal ultrasound scan may be an unexpected finding during a routine ultrasound scan or can be detected during a targeted ultrasound scan indicated by the finding of intrauterine fetal growth restriction, short long bones suggestive of a skeletal dysplasia, or other major fetal abnormalities. In these cases, the finding of limb abnormality can help in narrowing the differential diagnosis and directing additional investigation. Certain limb abnormalities can direct us toward a specific diagnosis: clenched hands in trisomy 18 and in other neurologic abnormalities, "hitchhiker" thumbs in diastrophic dysplasia, bent tibia and femur in camptomelic dysplasia, and sacral agenesis and absent/hypoplastic femurs in fetuses with diabetic embryopathy. Furthermore, the family history can indicate a recurrence when a limb abnormality is detected. Thus, thumb abnormality can indicate a recurrence in a family with a previous child with Fanconi's anemia and stippled epiphysis with a family history of chondrodysplasia punctata. When a limb abnormality is detected on fetal ultrasound scan, a referral should be made to a tertiary center with expertise in prenatal diagnosis of fetal anomalies. Fetal echocardiography should also be initiated. The approach should be multidisciplinary and include a medical geneticist, perinatologist, neonatologist, and fetal pathologist (if the pregnancy is being interrupted).

Etiologically, fetal limb abnormalities, as other abnormalities, can be divided into six categories:

1. Chromosome abnormalities (**Table 2**)
2. Single gene disorders (**Table 3**)
3. Multifactorial (**Box 1**)
4. Maternal diseases and exposures/teratogens (**Table 4**)

Detailed description of all types of limb abnormalities and the conditions associated with them is beyond the scope of this review. Some of the more common findings/diagnoses will thus be outlined. The nomenclature used in describing the type of limb abnormalities is outlined in **Table 1**.

MALFORMATION–DEFORMATION
Positional Abnormalities

Positional abnormalities can be classified as a deformation or a malformation. Thus, clubfeet can result from oligohydramnios or uterine septum and can also be the result of an abnormality in the formation of the feet. Positional abnormalities detected on fetal ultrasound scan include common abnormalities such as clinodactyly, camptodactyly, clenched fingers, and clubbed hands/feet. Almost all these conditions have a multifactorial mode of inheritance.

Clinodactyly

Clinodactyly is a fixed deviation of the fingers or toes. Clinodactyly of the toes is difficult to detect on fetal ultrasound scan; thus, the review concentrates on clinodactyly of the fingers. This abnormality affects each of the fingers but is most commonly seen as fifth finger clinodactyly. This abnormality results from asymmetrical hypoplasia

Table 3
Single gene disorders associated with limb abnormalities

Condition	Limb Abnormalities	Gene
Autosomal Dominant		
Holt Oram Syndrome	Upper limb only. Thumbs digitalized, absent, hypoplastic, triphalangeal, or, rarely, bifid; oligodactyly, syndactyly, and clinodactyly of fingers; limb reduction	TBX5
Okihiro syndrome	Thenar eminence hypoplasia, limitation in flexion of the first interphalangeal joint, absent, triphalangeal or hypoplastic thumbs, clubhand, spine abnormalities, lower limb abnormalities	SALL4
Cornelia de Lange	Micromelia, oligodactyly, limb reduction, clinodactyly of the fifth fingers, proximally placed thumbs, partial syndactyly of the second to third toes, limitation of elbow extension	NIPB1
Apert syndrome	Syndactyly of digits two through five and occasionally the thumbs—mitten hand (the fingernails might be fused), syndactyly of toes, preaxial polydactyly of the feet, short humeri, limited mobility of the shoulder and elbow joints.	FGFR2
Autosomal Recessive		
Fraser syndrome	Syndactyly of the fingers and toes	FRAS1, FREM2
Smith-Lemli-Opitz syndrome	Syndactyly of second to third toes, postaxial polydactyly	DHCR7
Fanconi pancytopenia	Thumb hypoplasia, triphalangeal/digitalized, supernumerary; clubhand; radial hypoplasia	FANC-A, C, D2, E, F, G and BRAC2
TAR syndrome	Radial aplasia with preservation of the thumbs, clubhand	Microdeletion 1q21.1
X-linked		
Goltz syndrome	Syndactyly of third to fourth fingers, polydactyly, ectrodactyly, oligodactyly, limb reduction	PORCN
Chondrodysplasia punctata - CDPX2	Stippled epiphyses, brachytelephalangy, short stature, rhizomelic shortening of the limbs	ARSE
Split-hand/foot malformation type 2	Syndactyly, median clefts of the hands and feet, aplasia or hypoplasia of the phalanges, metacarpals, and metatarsals	SHFM2
OPD (Oto-Palato-Digital) type I and II	Limited elbow and knee extension; radial head dislocation; mild lateral femoral bowing; short, broad distal phalanges, especially thumbs; short square nails; short third, fourth, and fifth metacarpals; supernumerary carpal bones; fusion of hamate and capitate; short, broad halluces toe syndactyly; anomalous fifth metatarsal; extra calcaneal ossification center; gap between first and second toes; dense long bones; radial, ulnar, femoral, and tibial bowing; small to absent fibula; subluxed elbow, wrist, and knee. Type II is allelic to type I but showed more severe findings including flexed overlapping fingers (trisomy 18–like); postaxial polydactyly and syndactyly of the fingers and toes; second finger clinodactyly; hypoplastic irregular metacarpals; short, broad hallucis; rockerbottom feet; "Tree-frog" hands and feet; hypoplastic metatarsals.	Filamin A gain of function mutations

> **Box 1**
> **Multifactorial conditions affecting the limbs**
>
> Congenital dislocation of the hips (CDH)
> Clubfeet
> Scoliosis

of the mid-phalanx with the medial part being shorter than the lateral part, resulting in radial angulation of the distal phalanx. In many cases, the clinodactyly is familial and isolated and has an autosomal dominant mode of inheritance with incomplete penetrance.[17] It is of utmost importance to recognize that clinodactyly exists in 18% of the normal population and has been reported in up to 60% of infants with Down syndrome. Thus, it is not a reliable sign for the detection of Down syndrome on fetal ultrasound scan when isolated.[18] However, when seen, other ultrasound findings suggestive of trisomy 21 should be looked for (thickened nuchal fold, heart defect, ventriculomegaly, hypoplastic nasal bone, short humerus and femur, and renal pelvis dilation).

Clubfeet

Clubfoot or talipes equinovarus is characterized by a foot fixed in adduction, supination, and varus position. There is subluxation of the talo-calcaneo-navicular joint, with underdevelopment of the soft tissues on the medial side of the foot and frequently of the calf and peroneal muscles.[19] As a result, the foot typically is turned inward, giving the foot a clublike appearance. This is one of the most common congenital birth defects and has been diagnosed as early as 13 weeks' gestation by transvaginal sonography[20,21] and at 16 weeks by transabdominal ultrasound scan.[22] Approximately one third of cases are isolated; however, many are associated with other abnormalities such as central nervous system abnormalities, the most common being neural tube defect. Thus, a thorough fetal ultrasound examination is important in prenatally diagnosed clubfeet (**Fig. 1**). The association of clubfeet with chromosome abnormality prompts the question of performing fetal karyotyping in isolated cases of clubfeet. In most cases of fetal chromosomal abnormalities, the clubfeet are not isolated. Because not all abnormalities are detectable by fetal ultrasound scan, fetal karyotyping should be offered.[23,24,25,26]

Clenched Hand

Clenched hand (the second and fifth fingers overlap the third and fourth with an adducted thumb) seen on fetal ultrasound scan must be evaluated carefully to determine that it is a persistent and not a temporary finding. When constant, it suggests the possibility of chromosomal abnormalities, particularly trisomy 18, as well as other causes of fetal akinesia sequence/arthrogryposis multiplex congenita. Both conditions are associated with poor prognosis (**Figs. 2 and 3**).[27,28]

Camptodactyly

Camptodactyly is a flexion contracture of one of the interphalangeal joints. Prenatally, only affected fingers can be diagnosed. Camptodactyly may be associated with chromosomal abnormalities, particularly when multiple fingers are affected (trisomy 18 and 13) as well as with inherited conditions such

Table 4
Maternal diseases and exposures associated with fetal limb abnormalities

Maternal Diseases and Teratogens Associated with Fetal Limb Abnormalities	Limb Abnormalities
Valproic Acid	Hypoplasia of distal phalanges
Carbamazepine	Hypoplasia of distal phalanges
Hydantoin	Hypoplasia of distal phalanges
Thalidomide	Limbs reduction
Imipramine	Limbs reduction (Amelia in one case)
Nortriptyline	Limb reduction defects (not confirmed)
Azathioprine	Preaxial polydactyly (not confirmed)
Cocaine	Limb reduction—vascular disruption
Maternal insulin-dependent diabetes mellitus	Sacral agenesis/femoral hypoplasia unusual face syndrome/caudal regression
Maternal autoimmune diseases	Chondrodysplasia punctata

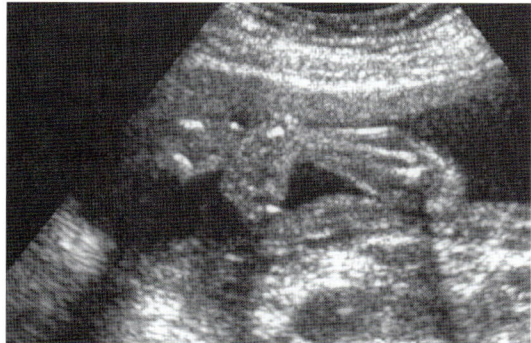

Fig. 1. Clubfoot. Foot has "hockey stick" configuration.

as Tel-Hashomer camptodactyly syndrome.[29] In many cases, it is part of a condition associated with arthrogryposis multiplex congenital, which can be a noninherited as in amyoplasia, or a variety of inherited conditions such as Larsen syndrome (autosomal recessive or dominant)[30] and geleophysic dysplasia (autosomal recessive).[31]

MALFORMATION–DISRUPTION
Abnormalities of Size and Number

This category includes abnormalities involving length or width. Abnormalities in width, such as macrodactyly, are known to be associated with conditions such as Proteus syndrome and are difficult to detect using fetal ultrasound scan. Length abnormalities are seen in different skeletal dysplasia and can be rhizomelic (short femurs or humeri), mesomelic (short forearms or calves), or acromelic (involving the hands or the feet). It is beyond the scope of this review to discuss the different types of skeletal dysplasia; therefore, this review focuses on isolated short long bones. These abnormalities can be caused by disruption, as in amniotic band sequence, or malformation, such as thalidomide teratogenicity.

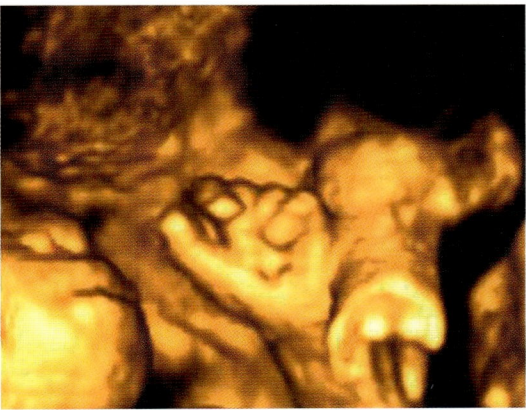

Fig. 2. Three-dimensional view of finger clenching in fetus with trisomy 18.

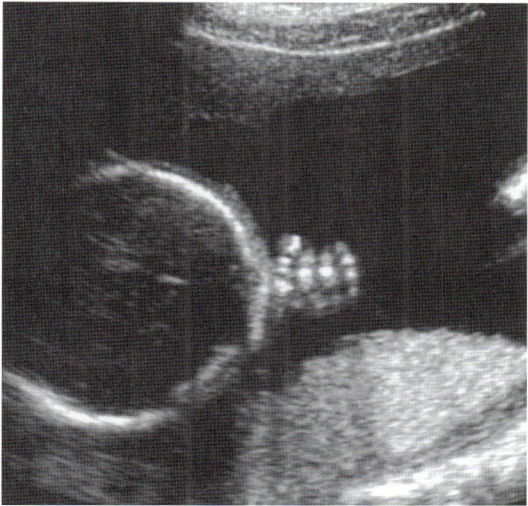

Fig. 3. Ultrasound scan shows finger clenching in fetus with trisomy 18.

Phocomelia

In phocomelia, the hands or feet are present, but the arms/forearms and thighs/calves are missing or foreshortened. The hands/feet may be normal or abnormal. The condition can be sporadic as well and associated with single gene disorders such as Robert syndrome, TAR (thrombocytopenia absent radius) syndrome, Grebe syndrome (see below) and teratogens such as thalidomide (**Fig 4**).[32]

Clubhand

This condition is divided into radial clubhand and ulnar clubhand. Radial and ulnar clubhand are frequently associated with radial ray and ulnar ray

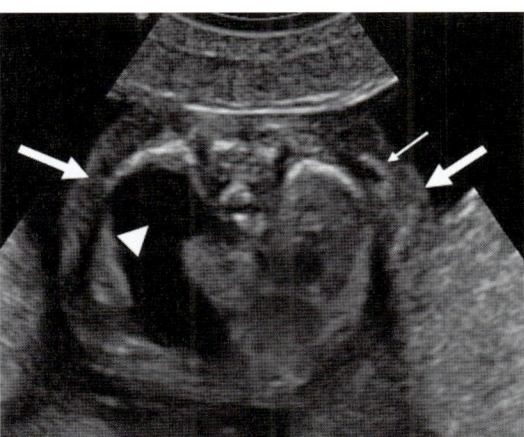

Fig. 4. Prenatal ultrasound scan of a fetus at 14 weeks with tetramelia and hydrops. *Thin arrow*, scapula; *thick arrows*, absent upper limbs; *arrowhead*, left pleural effusion.

Table 5
Conditions associated with radial ray defect

Condition	Other Manifestations
Autosomal recessive	
Rothmund-Thomson syndrome	Poikiloderma congenita, alopecia, photosensitivity, dystrophic nails, abnormal teeth, cataracts, short stature, and hypogonadism. Short and stubby hands and absent thumbs, eye abnormalities including iris dysgenesis, porokeratosis and cataracts, annular pancreas, duodenal stenosis. Thirty-two patients were screened for cataracts.
TAR syndrome	Bilateral absent radii but existent thumbs, ulnar and humeral hypoplasia, lower limb abnormalities have been reported but rare. Association with a submicroscopic deletion at 1q21.1 in some cases.
Fanconi anemia	IUGR; bone marrow failure; abnormalities of the eyes, kidneys, urinary tract, ear, heart, gastrointestinal system, oral cavity, and central nervous system; hearing loss; hypogonadism; developmental delay; and increased risk of malignancy. Genetically heterogenous.
Keutel syndrome	Microcephaly, occipital meningocele, dysplastic ears, optic atrophy, vertebral abnormalities, limb problems including radiohumeral synostosis, subluxation of one hip, joint contractures, and focal femoral hypoplasia.
Roberts and/or SC phocomelia syndrome	IUGR, tetraphocomelia, or hypomelia caused by mesomelic shortening of the limbs with radial defects and oligodactyly or syndactyly (the upper limbs are more severely affected than lower limbs), cleft lip/palate, large genitalia, congenital heart defects, cystic kidneys, characteristic face with hypertelorism, a prominent premaxilla, a mid-face capillary hemangioma, cloudy corneas or cataracts and dysplastic or small ears, micrognathia, beaked nose, ear malformations, and mental retardation
Autosomal Dominant	
Diamond-Blackfan syndrome	Developmental delay, triphalangeal thumbs, hypoplastic anemia, hypertelorism, retinopathy, cleft palate, short webbed neck, parietal foramina, scoliosis.
Holt-Oram syndrome	Cardiac abnormalities including atrial septal defect (ostium secundum type), ventricular septal defect, hypoplastic left heart, and patent ductus arteriosus. Upper limb abnormalities can be asymmetrical and include absent, bifid, or triphalangeal thumbs; carpal bone anomalies; phocomelia; and radial-ulnar anomalies
Okihiro syndrome	Uni- or bilateral radial ray malformation including thenar hypoplasia, thumb hypoplasia/aplasia, triphalangeal, preaxial polydactyly, clubhand, deviation of the forearms, Duane anomaly, sensorineural or conductive deafness, and renal abnormalities
de Lange syndrome	Upper limb reduction defects ranging from subtle phalangeal abnormalities to oligodactyly, IUGR, micrognathia, cardiac abnormalities, microcephaly, and ambiguous genitalia

Chromosomal abnormalities	
Trisomy 13	Profound mental retardation, scalp defects, holoprosencephaly, sloping forehead, anophthalmia/microphthalmia, absent nose, cyclopia, proboscis, bulbous nose, cleft lip/palate, cardiac abnormalities, omphalocele, ambiguous genitalia, postaxial polydactyly, neural tube defects
Trisomy 18	IUGR; microcephaly; choroid plexus cysts; facial dysmorphism; cleft lip; micrognathia; ear, nose, and throat abnormalities; cataract, microphthalmia cardiac anomalies; diaphragmatic hernia; omphalocele; clenched hand; clubhand; rocker bottom feet; prominent heels
Teratogens	
Thalidomide embryopathy	Limb abnormalities including phocomelia, amelia, clubfeet, polydactyly, microtia, facial palsy, orofacial cleft, microphthalmia, cardiac defect, IUGR, urogenital, gastrointestinal, and spinal defects
Varicella embryopathy	IUGR, clubfeet, abnormal position of the hands, limitation of limb extension, limb hypoplasia, chorioretinitis, cataracts, microphthalmia, microcephaly
Others	
Klippel-Feil syndrome	Cervical vertebral fusions, microtia, conductive deafness, restriction of supination of the forearms, thenar hypoplasia, thumb hypoplasia, radial aplasia, absence of metacarpals, humerus, and ulnar hypoplasia. Unknown inheritance
VACTERL association	Vertebral defects, anal atresia/stenosis, cardiac abnormalities, tracheo-esophageal fistula/esophageal atresia, radial and other limb defects, and renal anomalies

Abbreviation: IUGR, intrauterine growth restriction.

abnormalities, respectively.[32–34] Radial clubhand is the more common abnormality detected prenatally and in most cases is associated with other abnormalities, many of them inherited (**Table 5**).

Ulnar clubhand is secondary to ulnar ray deficiency. This is a rare anomaly and is usually nonsyndromic, although it can occur in association with conditions such as Larsen syndrome or TAU syndrome (thrombocytopenia and absent ulna with mental retardation and facial dysmorphism).[35] The condition may be associated with skeletal dysplasia and arthrogryposis. Prenatal differentiation between ulnar clubhand and radial clubhand is difficult, and in many cases ulnar clubhand is associated with a radial ray defect also (**Figs. 5–7**).

Thumb Anomalies

Thumb anomalies deserve special attention in view of the important differential diagnosis associated with these conditions (see **Table 5**). The prenatal diagnosis of thumb abnormalities includes thumb hypoplasia, triphalangeal thumb, broad thumb, and hitchhiker thumb. Thumb abnormalities may be isolated but in most cases are associated with other body organ or limb abnormalities. The extremely rare hitchhiker thumb deformation corresponds to the abnormally abducted position of a more proximally inserted thumb.[32,36,37] This constant malposition is suggestive of diastrophic dysplasia, a rare skeletal dysplasia with an autosomal recessive mode of inheritance that is amenable to prenatal diagnosis.[32,36,37]

Polydactyly

Polydactyly is frequently detected using fetal ultrasound scan as the presence of extra digit/s in the

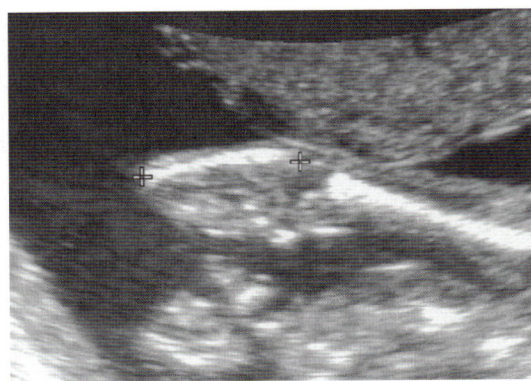

Fig. 6. Clubhand. Humerus is normal. Forearm has single short bone. Hand and wrist are flexed acutely and lie along anterior aspect of forearm. Fetus has trisomy 18.

upper or lower extremities. The extra digits may vary in their developmental maturity. The extra digit can appear on the radial side (preaxial) or on the ulnar side (postaxial) polydactyly. Meso-axial polydactyly is less frequent than pre-/postaxial polydactyly. Postaxial polydactyly is more frequent than preaxial polydactyly, particularly among Africans. The incidence of polydactyly is one in 700 pregnancies.[38] Postaxial polydactyly can be an isolated finding, usually with an autosomal dominant mode of inheritance with incomplete penetrance or part of a syndrome. Several familial

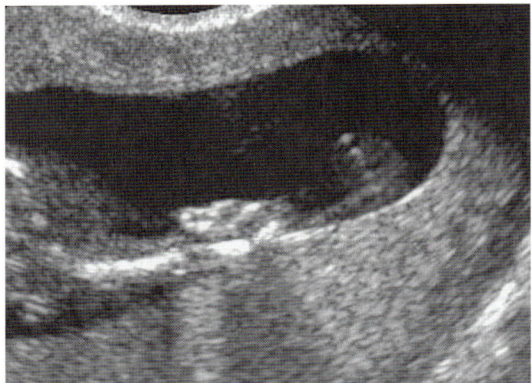

Fig. 5. Clubhand. Humerus adjacent to fetal trunk is normal. Hand and fingers are markedly flexed at wrist and lie along forearm.

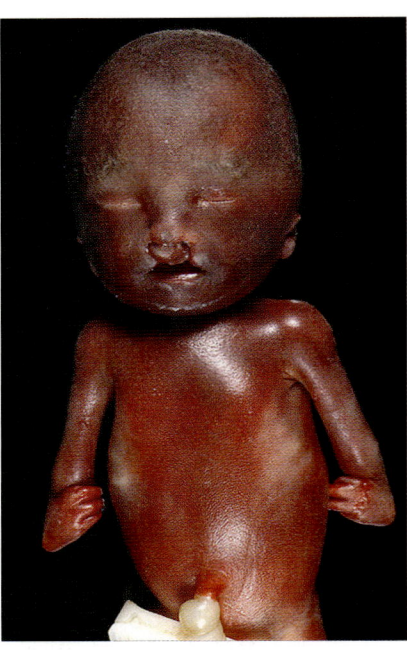

Fig. 7. Bilateral clubhands. Forearms are short. Hands are acutely flexed at wrists and only three digits. Also bilateral cleft lip.

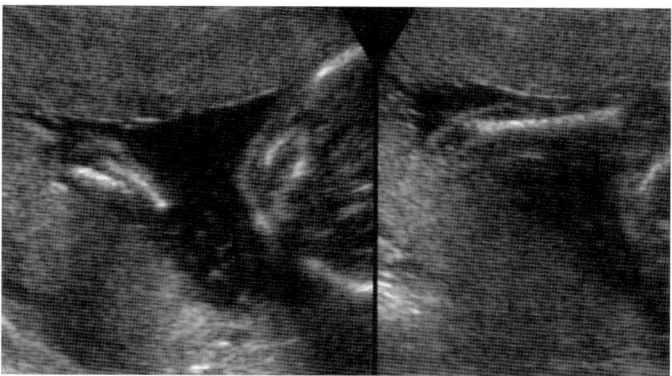

Fig. 8. Forearm amputation. Left image shows radius and ulna amputated at mid-forearm. Right image shows normal humerus.

cases of mutations in the GLI3 gene mapping to 7p13[39] have been as well as other genes reported.

Preaxial polydactyly is a highly variable condition ranging from broad thumb to duplication of the thumb and can be isolated (autosomal dominant) or part of a syndrome. Mutations of regulatory genes affecting the SHH pathway[40] have been reported in some families with isolated preaxial polydactyly.

Terminal Transverse Limb Defects

Generally, terminal transverse defects are more common in the upper limbs than the lower limbs; they may be isolated or part of syndromes and are likely to be associated with other abnormalities. The condition is thought to result from a vascular injury and has been found in association with coagulation defects[13] as well as conditions causing fetal hypoxemia, such as α-thalassemia homozygous state,[41] or after chorionic villus sampling.[42] In many cases the condition is the result of constriction band sequence/amniotic band sequence, caused by early rupture of the amnion and formation of fibrous bands that can trap, constrict, and disrupt fetal parts. The presentation can vary from a simple circumferential groove to ring constriction, amputation of part of a finger resulting in whole-limb amputation, or severe malformations including syndactyly, pterygium, and lethal craniofacial or thoraco-abdominal destructive possesses. Disruptions caused by amniotic bands are characteristically asymmetrical and are amenable to ultrasound detection, but the wide range of abnormalities makes the diagnosis challenging. The differential diagnosis of this condition includes Adams-Oliver syndrome (aplasia cutis congenita, limb defects)[43] with an autosomal dominant mode of inheritance (**Figs. 8** and **9**).

Ectrodactyly (Split Hand/Split Foot)

Split hand/foot deformity, also known as lobster claw hand/foot, results from a deficiency of the central digits/toes with a deep V- or U-shaped central cleft. The main pathogenic mechanism is most probably a failure of the median apical

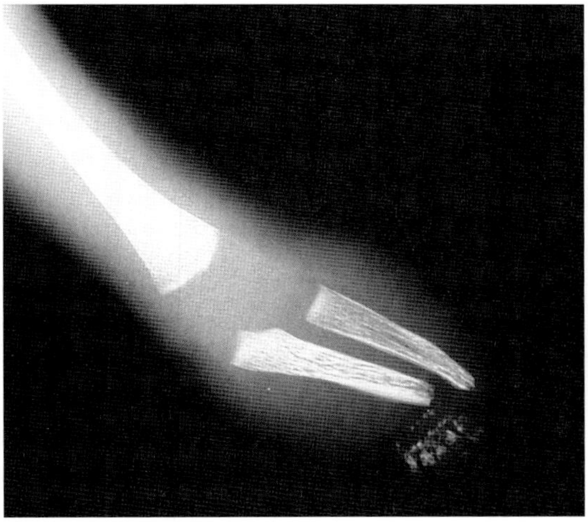

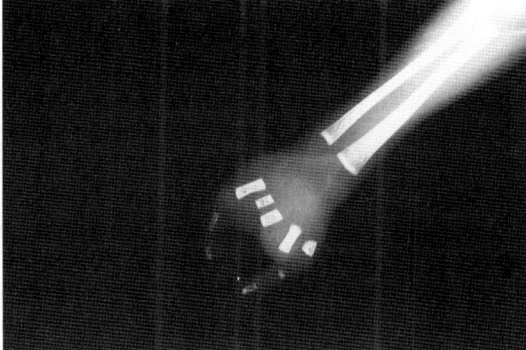

Fig. 10. Ectrodactyly X-ray. Only thumb and little finger have phalanges, and these are abnormal. Middle three metacarpals are short, and phalanges are missing.

Fig. 9. X-ray of arm amputation at mid-forarm.

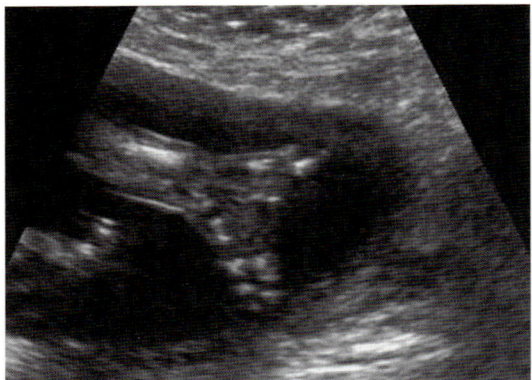

Fig. 11. Ectrodactyly on ultrasound scan at 20 weeks. Hand has a V-deformity with thumb on one side and two fingers with syndactyly on the other. Middle metacarpals and phalanges are missing.

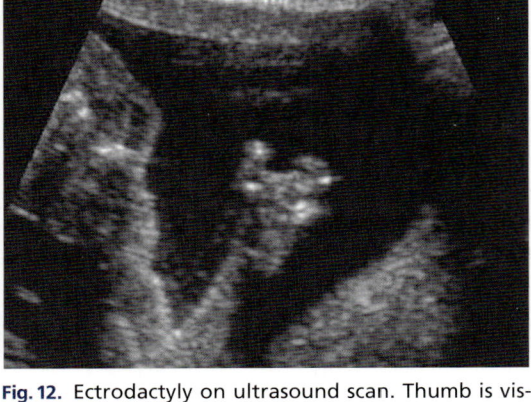

Fig. 12. Ectrodactyly on ultrasound scan. Thumb is visible on one side of the V defect. Malformed fingers on the other side.

ectodermal ridge in the developing limb bud.[44] It may be isolated or associated with other abnormalities such as in EEC syndrome (ectrodactyly, ectodermal dysplasia, cleft lip/palate) and syndactyly, absence, or hypoplasia of the residual phalanges; metacarpals/metatarsal can also be seen (**Figs. 10–12**). The severity of the malformation is variable, and the inheritance can be autosomal recessive, autosomal dominant, or X-linked.[45]

Syndactyly

Syndactyly is a condition in which two or more digits are fused together. It is the most common congenital malformation of the limbs, with an incidence of 1 in 2000 to 3000 live births.[46,47] The condition is the result of failure of separation of the fingers or toes into individual appendages, which usually occurs between the sixth and seventh week postconception.

Syndactyly is defined as *simple* when it involves soft tissue only or *complex* when it involves the bone or nail of the adjacent fingers or toes that are joined side by side. It can be complete when the fusion extends to the tip of the finger or toe or incomplete when the soft-tissue union does not extend to the fingertips. Complex syndactyly refers to fingers joined by bone or cartilaginous union, usually in a side-to-side fashion at the distal phalanges. The most severe form of syndactyly is classified as complicated syndactyly which refers to fingers joined by bony fusion other than a side-to-side and can include bony abnormalities such as extra, missing, or duplicated phalanges and abnormally shaped bones such as delta phalanges. The complex type of syndactyly may be associated with other finger or toe abnormalities including polydactyly, oligodactyly, or duplicated phalanges as well as abnormally shaped bones. The condition can be an isolated finding or associated with other abnormalities, and more than 30 syndromes with syndactyly have been reported,

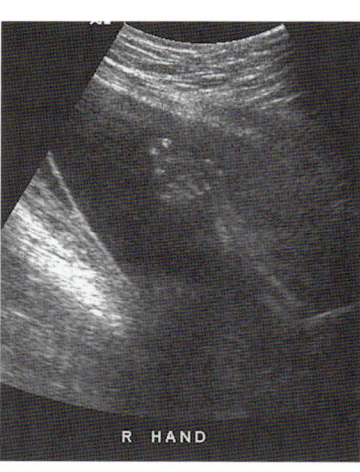
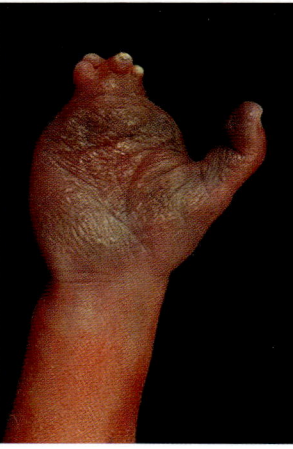

Fig. 13. Fetal ultrasound scan and autopsy show complex, complete syndactyly.

including Poland, Apert, Fraser and Holt-Oram syndromes. Simple syndactyly is more common between the third and fourth fingers and the second and third toes. In 50% of the cases it is bilateral.

Prenatal diagnosis of simple toe syndactyly is almost impossible, whereas prenatal diagnosis of finger simple syndactyly is possible but very challenging. The diagnosis is easier when the syndactyly is complete and complex because it is associated with bony changes in shape and results in synchronous movements of the affected digits. In cases of mitten hand deformity as seen in Apert syndrome, the fingers and toes cannot be seen individually, which makes the prenatal diagnosis easier (**Fig. 13**).[48]

SUMMARY

The detection of fetal limb abnormalities, using ultrasonography, is of utmost importance for prenatal diagnosis of fetal anomalies and for providing accurate genetic counseling. Limb abnormalities may be isolated or associated with other abnormalities and can be the result of malformation, deformation, or disruption, as well as part of a dysplasia such as skeletal dysplasia. When the limb anomaly is a malformation and associated with other abnormalities, it is usually the result of a chromosomal abnormality or single gene disorder. The prenatal diagnosis and management of limb abnormalities is complex and requires a multidisciplinary approach of radiologists, perinatologists, medical geneticists, neonatologists, and orthopedic surgeons to provide the couple/woman with information regarding the nature of the abnormality, differential diagnosis, prognosis, and options related to the pregnancy.

REFERENCES

1. Johnson J-AM. Overview of obstetric sonography. In: Rumack CM, Wilson SR, Charboneau JW, editors. Diagnostic Ultrasound. 3rd edition. St. Louis, MO: Elsevier; 2005. p. 1039–58.
2. Gramellini D, Fieni S, Vadora E. Prenatal diagnosis of isolated limb defects: an updated review. Fetal Diagn Ther 2005;20(2):96–101.
3. Bavinck JN, Weaver DD. Subclavian artery supply disruption sequence: hypothesis of a vascular etiology for Poland, Klippel-Feil, and Mobius anomalies. Am J Med Genet 1986;23(4):903–18.
4. Kleist-Retzow JC, Cormier-Daire V, Viot G, et al. Antenatal manifestations of mitochondrial respiratory chain deficiency. J Pediatr 2003;143(2):208–12.
5. Mittal TK, Vujanic GM, Morrissey BM, et al. Triploidy: antenatal sonographic features with post-mortem correlation. Prenat Diagn 1998;18(12):1253–62.
6. le Vaillant C, Quere MP, David A, et al. Prenatal diagnosis of a 'minor' form of Brachmann-de Lange syndrome by three-dimensional sonography and three-dimensional computed tomography. Fetal Diagn Ther 2004;19(2):155–9.
7. Emanuel PG, Garcia GI, Angtuaco TL. Prenatal detection of anterior abdominal wall defects with US. Radiographics 1995;15(3):517–30.
8. Espinasse M, Manouvrier S, Boute O, et al. [Embryofetopathy due to valproate: a pathology only little known. Apropos of 4 cases]. Arch Pediatr 1996;3(9):896–9 [French].
9. Holder-Espinasse M, Devisme L, Thomas D, et al. Pre- and postnatal diagnosis of limb anomalies: a series of 107 cases. Am J Med Genet A 2004;124A(4):417–22.
10. Pauli RM, Lebovitz RM, Meyer RD. Familial recurrence of terminal transverse defects of the arm. Clin Genet 1985;27(6):555–63.
11. Pilarski RT, Pauli RM, Engber WD. Hand-reduction malformations: genetic and syndromic analysis. J Pediatr Orthop 1985;5(3):274–80.
12. Froster UG, Baird PA. Amniotic band sequence and limb defects: data from a population-based study. Am J Med Genet 1993;46(5):497–500.
13. Hunter AG. A pilot study of the possible role of familial defects in anticoagulation as a cause for terminal limb reduction malformations. Clin Genet 2000;57(3):197–204.
14. Sabry MA, Obenbergerova D, Al Sawan R, et al. Femoral hypoplasia-unusual facies syndrome with bifid hallux, absent tibia, and macrophallus: a report of a Bedouin baby. J Med Genet 1996;33(2):165–7.
15. Rodriguez-Pinilla E, Arroyo I, Fondevilla J, et al. Prenatal exposure to valproic acid during pregnancy and limb deficiencies: a case-control study. Am J Med Genet 2000;90(5):376–81.
16. Stoll C, Calzolari E, Cornel M, et al. A study on limb reduction defects in six European regions. Ann Genet 1996;39(2):99–104.
17. Kozin SH. Upper-extremity congenital anomalies. J Bone Joint Surg Am 2003;85-A(8):1564–76.
18. Budorick N. The fetal musculoskeletal system. In: Callen P, editor. Ultrasonography in obstetrics and gynecology. Philadelphia: Saunders WB; 2000. p. 331–77.
19. Drvaric DM, Kuivila TE, Roberts JM. Congenital clubfoot. Etiology, pathoanatomy, pathogenesis, and the changing spectrum of early management. Orthop Clin North Am 1989;20(4):641–7.
20. Bar-Hava I, Bronshtein M, Orvieto R, et al. Caution: prenatal clubfoot can be both a transient and a late-onset phenomenon. Prenat Diagn 1997;17(5):457–60.
21. Bronshtein M, Zimmer EZ. Transvaginal ultrasound diagnosis of fetal clubfeet at 13 weeks, menstrual age. J Clin Ultrasound 1989;17(7):518–20.

22. Benacerraf BR. Antenatal sonographic diagnosis of congenital clubfoot: a possible indication for amniocentesis. J Clin Ultrasound 1986;14(9):703–6.
23. Canto MJ, Cano S, Palau J, et al. Prenatal diagnosis of clubfoot in low-risk population: associated anomalies and long-term outcome. Prenat Diagn 2008; 28(4):343–6.
24. Malone FD, Marino T, Bianchi DW, et al. Isolated clubfoot diagnosed prenatally: is karyotyping indicated? Obstet Gynecol 2000;95(3):437–40.
25. Mammen L, Benson CB. Outcome of fetuses with clubfeet diagnosed by prenatal sonography. J Ultrasound Med 2004;23(4):497–500.
26. Woodrow N, Tran T, Umstad M, et al. Mid-trimester ultrasound diagnosis of isolated talipes equinovarus: accuracy and outcome for infants. Aust N Z J Obstet Gynaecol 1998;38(3):301–5.
27. Ryu JK, Cho JY, Choi JS. Prenatal sonographic diagnosis of focal musculoskeletal anomalies. Korean J Radiol 2003;4(4):243–51.
28. Tongsong T, Sirichotiyakul S, Wanapirak C, et al. Sonographic features of trisomy 18 at midpregnancy. J Obstet Gynaecol Res 2002;28(5):245–50.
29. Franceschini P, Vardeu MP, Signorile F, et al. Inguinal hernia and atrial septal defect in Tel Hashomer camptodactyly syndrome: report of a new case expanding the phenotypic spectrum of the disease. Am J Med Genet 1993;46(3):341–4.
30. Bicknell LS, Farrington-Rock C, Shafeghati Y, et al. A molecular and clinical study of Larsen syndrome caused by mutations in FLNB. J Med Genet 2007; 44(2):89–98.
31. Wraith JE, Bankier A, Chow CW, et al. Geleophysic dysplasia. Am J Med Genet 1990;35(2):153–6.
32. Taybi H, Lachman R. Radiology of syndromes, metabolic disorders and skeletal dysplasias. 5th edition. St. Louis, MO: Mosby; 1996.
33. James MA, McCarroll HR Jr, Manske PR. The spectrum of radial longitudinal deficiency: a modified classification. J Hand Surg [Am] 1999;24(6):1145–55.
34. Romero R, Athanassiadis AP, Jeanty P. Fetal skeletal anomalies. Radiol Clin North Am 1990;28(1):75–99.
35. Stoll C, Finck S, Janser B, et al. Tau syndrome (thrombocytopenia and absent ulnar) with mental retardation and facial dysmorphy. Genet Couns 1992; 3(1):41–7.
36. Tongsong T, Wanapirak C, Sirichotiyakul S, et al. Prenatal sonographic diagnosis of diastrophic dwarfism. J Clin Ultrasound 2002;30(2):103–5.
37. Wax JR, Carpenter M, Smith W, et al. Second-trimester sonographic diagnosis of diastrophic dysplasia: report of 2 index cases. J Ultrasound Med 2003; 22(8):805–8.
38. Teot L, Deschamps F. [Histologic and echographic correlations of the hip in newborn infants]. Rev Chir Orthop Reparatrice Appar Mot 1990;76(1):8–16 [French].
39. Richards DS. Complications of prolonged PROM and oligohydramnios. Clin Obstet Gynecol 1998; 41(4):817–26.
40. Usta IM, AbuMusa AA, Khoury NG, et al. Early ultrasonographic changes in Fowler syndrome features and review of the literature. Prenat Diagn 2005; 25(11):1019–23.
41. Chitayat D, Silver MM, O'Brien K, et al. Limb defects in homozygous alpha-thalassemia: report of three cases. Am J Med Genet 1997;68(2):162–7.
42. Golden CM, Ryan LM, Holmes LB. Chorionic villus sampling: a distinctive teratogenic effect on fingers? Birth Defects Res A Clin Mol Teratol 2003;67(8): 557–62.
43. Verdyck P, Holder-Espinasse M, Hul WV, et al. Clinical and molecular analysis of nine families with Adams-Oliver syndrome. Eur J Hum Genet 2003; 11(6):457–63.
44. Duijf PH, van Bokhoven H, Brunner HG. Pathogenesis of split-hand/split-foot malformation. Hum Mol Genet 2003;(12 Spec No 1):R51–60.
45. Elliott AM, Evans JA, Chudley AE. Split hand foot malformation (SHFM). Clin Genet 2005;68(6): 501–5.
46. Lamb DW, Wynne-Davies R, Soto L. An estimate of the population frequency of congenital malformations of the upper limb. J Hand Surg [Am] 1982; 7(6):557–62.
47. Light TR. Congenital anomalies: syndactyly, polydactyly and cleft hand. In: Peimer CA, editor. Surgery of the hand and upper extremity. New York: McGraw-Hill; 1996. p. 2111–44.
48. Skidmore DL, Pai AP, Toi A, et al. Prenatal diagnosis of Apert syndrome: report of two cases. Prenat Diagn 2003;23(12):1009–13.

Index

Note: Page numbers of article titles are in **boldface** type.

A

Acrania, 589
Acrocephalosyndactyly, 586
Amniotic bands, 605–606
Amputations, prenatal, 605–606
Anencephaly, 531–532, 589
Angiography, 524
Angiotensin-converting enzyme inhibitors, fetopathy due to, 591
Antley-Bixler syndrome, 586
Apert syndrome, 586, 599
Arachnoid cysts, 505, 507–508, 510–511, 553–554
Arteriovenous fistulas, 571–572
Association, definition of, 596

B

Baller-Gerold syndrome, 586
"Banana sign," in spina bifida, 535, 587–588
Biparietal diameter, 583–584
Blake's pouch cyst, persistent, 514
Brachycephaly, 583, 585, 587
Brain anomalies. *See also specific anomalies.*
    cranial imaging in, **583–594**
    cystic, **553–558**
    magnetic resonance imaging in, **559–582**
    neural migration, **541–552**
    three-dimensional scan in, **489–528**

C

Camptodactyly, 601
Carpenter syndrome, 586
Cephalic index, 583–584
Cephaloceles, 504–507, 569, 588–589
Cerebellum
    hemorrhage of, 576
    hypoplasia of, 575–576
Cerebral cortex
    abnormal neuron migration to, 542–551, 565–569
    normal development of, 541–543
Chiari malformations, 569, 576–577
Chondrodysplasia punctata, 599
Choroid plexus cysts, 556–557
Choroid plexus papillomas, 556
Cisterna magna, enlarged, 514–515
Clenched hand, 600
Cloverleaf skull, 585, 587
Clubfoot, 600
Clubhand, 601, 604
Colpocephaly, 563–564
Cornelia de Lange syndrome, 599, 602
Corpus callosum agenesis, 498–503, 563–565
Cranial ultrasound. *See* Skull ultrasound.
Craniopharyngiomas, 577–578
Craniosynostosis, 585–587
Crouzon syndrome, 586
Cyst(s), **553–558**
    arachnoid, 505, 507–508, 510–511, 553–554
    Blake's pouch, 514
    choroid plexus, 556–557
    endodermal, 554
    intraparenchymal, 555–556
    intraventricular, 556–557
    neuroectodermal, 554
    of extra-axial origin, 553–555
    porencephalic, 554, 556
Cytomegalovirus infections, 578

D

Dandy-Walker malformation, 512–513, 574–575
Dandy-Walker variant, 513–514, 574–575
Deformations, 596, 598, 600–601
Diamond-Blackfan syndrome, 602
Digital abnormalities
    camptodactyly, 601
    clenched hand, 600
    clinodactyly, 598, 600
    clubhand, 601, 604
    ectrodactyly, 606
    polydactyly, 604–605
    syndactyly, 605–606
    thumb, 604
Disruptions, 596, 601–607
Dolichocephaly, 583, 585
Dural arteriovenous fistulas, 571–572
Dysplasia, definition of, 596
Dysraphism, spinal, occult, 537–538

Index

E

Ectrodactyly, 599, 606
Encephaloceles, 505, 532–534, 588–589
Endodermal cysts, 554

F

Fanconi syndrome, 599, 602
Fetal limb abnormalities, **595–608**
Fetal neuroimaging
    in brain anomalies, magnetic resonance imaging
        after, **559–582**
    in cranial anomalies, **583–594**
    in intracranial cystic lesions, **553–558**
    in neural migration disorders, **541–552**
    in spinal abnormalities, **529–539**
    three-dimensional, **489–528**
        advantages of, 524–525
        display modalities for, 518–524
        in angiography, 524
        in arachnoid cyst, 505, 507–508, 510–511
        in cephalocele, 504–507
        in corpus callosum agenesis, 498–503
        in holoprosencephaly, 503–504
        in posterior fossa anomalies, 509–515
        in skull abnormalities, 591–592
        limitations of, 526–527
        procedure for, 489–501
        technical aspects of, 517–518
Finger abnormalities. *See* Digital abnormalities.
Foot, club, 600
Fraser syndrome, 599

G

Germinal matrix hemorrhage, 571–572
Glioependymal cysts, 554–555
Gliomas, 577–578
Goodman syndrome, 586

H

Hand
    clenched, 600
    club, 601, 604
Head circumference, measurement of, 583–585
Hemimegalencephaly, 566
Hemivertebrae, 535–536
Hemorrhage, brain, 571–572
Heterotopia, 567–568
Hitchhiker thumb, 604
Holoprosencephaly, 503–504, 569–571
Holt-Oram syndrome, 599, 602
Hydrocephalus, 521–522, 554
Hypophosphatasia, 591
Hypoxia, cerebral ischemia in, 572–573

I

Infections, 578
Intraparenchymal cysts, 555–556
Intraventricular cysts, 556–557
Ischemia, cerebral, 572–573

J

Jackson-Weiss syndrome, 586

K

Keutel syndrome, 602
Kleeblattschädel, 585, 587
Klippel-Feil syndrome, 603

L

Larsen syndrome, 601, 604
"Lemon sign"
    in cephaloceles, 589
    in spina bifida, 587–588
Leukomalacia, periventricular, 555–556
Limb abnormalities, **595–608**
    camptodactyly, 601
    clenched hand, 600
    clinodactyly, 598, 600
    clubfeet, 600
    clubhand, 601
    conditions associated with, 596
    definitions of, 596
    differential diagnosis of, 598
    ectrodactytly, 599, 606
    embryology of, 595
    etiologies of, 598
    lissencephaly, 544, 548–551
    phocomelia, 601
    polydactyly, 604–605
    positional, 598
    prevalence of, 595
    radial ray defects, 602–603
    single-gene, 599
    stepwise approach to, 595–598
    syndactyly, 606–607
    terminal transverse, 605–606
    terminology of, 596–597
    thumb, 604
Lissencephaly
    cerebellar hypoplasia with, 544
    classic type, 544, 549, 566–567
    classification of, 544
    cobblestone type, 544, 550–551
    microcephaly with, 544
    X-linked, 544
Lobster claw syndrome, 599, 606

M

Magnetic resonance imaging, **559–582**
  in callosal agenesis, 563–565
  in cephalocele, 569
  in cortical abnormalities, 565–569
  in hemimegalencephaly, 566
  in hemorrhage, 571–572
  in heterotopia, 567–568
  in holoprosencephaly, 569–571
  in infections, 578
  in lissencephaly, 566–567
  in microlissencephaly, 566
  in muscular dystrophy, 568–569
  in neoplasia, 577–578
  in neural migration disorders, 565–569
  in normal brain, 561
  in polymicrogyria, 568
  in posterior fossa abnormalities, 573–577
  in schizencephaly, 566
  in twin-twin transfusion, 572–573
  in vascular insults, 572–573
  in vascular malformations, 571–572
  in ventriculomegaly, 561–563
  limitations of, 560
  safety of, 560–561
  technique for, 560
Malformations, 596, 598–607
Meckel-Gruber syndrome, 589
Mega cisterna magna, 514–515
Meningoceles, 505–507, 533–534
Microcephaly, 589–590
Microlissencephaly, 566
Miller-Dieker syndrome, 544, 567
Muscular dystrophy, congenital, 568–569
Myelomeningoceles, 534, 576–577

N

Nasal bone length, 584
Neoplasia, congenital, 577–578
Neural migration disorders, **541–552**
  focal, 542–543, 545–547
  lissencephaly, 544–551
  schizencephaly, 551
  types of, 543
  versus normal cortical development, 541–543
Neural tube defects, 530–535, 587–589
Neuroectodermal cysts, 554–555
Neuroimaging, fetal. *See* Fetal neuroimaging.
Norman-Roberts syndrome, 544

O

Okihiro syndrome, 599, 602
Opitz syndrome, 586
Ossification, skull, abnormal, 591
Osteogenesis imperfecta, 590–591
Oto-palato-digital syndrome, 599
Oxycephaly, 585

P

Pachygyria, 544, 548, 566–567
Papillomas, choroid plexus, 556
Periventricular pseudocysts, 555–556
Pfeiffer syndrome, 586
Phocomelia, 601–602
Plagiocephaly, 585
Polydactyly, 604–605
Polymicrogyria, 568
Porencephalic cysts, 554, 556
Posterior fossa abnormalities, 509–515, 573–577

R

Roberts phocomelia syndrome, 602
Rothmund-Thomson syndrome, 602

S

Saethre-Chotzen syndrome, 586
Sakati-Nyhan syndrome, 586
Scaphocephaly, 583
Schizencephaly, 551, 566
Sequence, definition of, 596
Shprintzen-Goldberg syndrome, 586
Skull ultrasound, **583–594**
  in craniosynostosis, 585–587
  in microcephaly, 589–590
  in neural tube defects, 587–589
  in osteogenesis imperfecta, 590–591
  in shape variations, 583–585
  normal, 583–585
  three-dimensional, 591–592
Smith-Lemli-Opitz syndrome, 599
Spina bifida, 532, 534–535, 587–588
Spinal anomalies, **529–539**
  hemivertebrae, 535–536
  imaging technique for, 529–531
  neural tube defects, 530–535
  occult dysraphism, 537–538
  tethered spinal cord, 537–538
Split-hand/foot syndrome, 599, 606
"Steer's horns" appearance, in corpus callosum agenesis, 563–564
Strawberry-shaped skull, 587
"Sunburst sign," in corpus callosum agenesis, 502
Sutures, premature fusion of (craniosynostosis), 585–587
Syndactyly, 606–607
Syndrome, definition of, 596
Syntelencephaly, 570–571

T

Talipes equinovarus, 600
TAR syndrome, 599, 602, 604
Tel-Hashomer syndrome, 601
Teratogens, limb abnormalities due to, 603
Teratomas, 577–578
Terminal transverse limb defects, 605–606
Tethered spinal cord, 537–538
Thalidomide embryopathy, 603
Thumb anomalies, 604
Toes, abnormalities of. *See* Digital abnormalities.
TORCH infections, 578
Toxoplasmosis, 578
Transmantle cortical dysplasia with balloon cells, 565–566
Trigonocephaly, 585
Trisomy 13, 603
Trisomy 18, 603
Tuberous sclerosis, cortical dysplasia in, 565–566
Turricephaly, 585
Twin-twin transfusion, 572–573

U

Ulnar clubhand, 600, 604

V

VACTERL association, 535–536, 603
Varicella embryopathy, 603
Vascular malformations, 571–572
Vein of Galen malformations, 571–572
Ventriculomegaly, magnetic resonance imaging, 561–563
Vertebral anomalies, 535–536
"Viking's helmet sign," in corpus callosum agenesis, 502

W

Walker-Warburg syndrome, 532, 544, 568–569, 589

X

X-linked syndromes, limb abnormalities in, 599